Grassroots Medicine

Grassroots Medicine

The Story of America's Free Health Clinics

Gregory L. Weiss

ROWMAN & LITTLEFIELD PUBLISHERS, INC.
Lanham • Boulder • New York • Toronto • Oxford

ROWMAN & LITTLEFIELD PUBLISHERS, INC.

Published in the United States of America
by Rowman & Littlefield Publishers, Inc.
A wholly owned subsidiary of The Rowman & Littlefield Publishing Group, Inc.
4501 Forbes Boulevard, Suite 200, Lanham, Maryland 20706
www.rowmanlittlefield.com

P.O. Box 317, Oxford OX2 9RU, UK

British Library Cataloguing in Publication Information Available

Library of Congress Cataloging-in-Publication Data
Weiss, Gregory L.
  Grassroots medicine : the story of America's free health clinics / Gregory L. Weiss.
    p. ; cm.
  Includes bibliographical references and index.
  ISBN-13: 978-0-7425-4069-9 (cloth : alk. paper)
  ISBN-10: 0-7425-4069-3 (cloth : alk. paper)
  ISBN-13: 978-0-7425-4070-5 (pbk. : alk. paper)
  ISBN-10: 0-7425-4070-7 (pbk. : alk. paper)
  1. Clinics. 2. Community health services. 3. Health facilities. 4. Hospitals. I.
Title. [DNLM: 1. Community Health Services—United States. 2. Community
Health Centers—United States. 3. Health Services Accessibility—United States. 4.
Medically Uninsured—United States. WA 546 AA1 W429g 2005]
  RA965.W45 2006
  362.12—dc22

                                                                  2005021101

Printed in the United States of America

⊗™ The paper used in this publication meets the minimum requirements of
American National Standard for Information Sciences—Permanence of Paper
for Printed Library Materials, ANSI/NISO Z39.48-1992.

To Robert Eichhorn, who introduced me to medical sociology

To Estelle Nichols Avner, who introduced me to free clinics

and

To the tens of thousands of professional and lay volunteers
in free health clinics throughout the United States

Contents

Preface

While I was in graduate school at Purdue University in the early 1970s, my advisor, Robert Eichhorn, shared with me his interest in the inability of many low-income individuals and families to access private care. This was especially significant at this particular time. Medicaid had been passed in 1965 and had gone into effect in 1966, and early analysis of data showed that the number of physician visits by the poor had increased. There was some early optimism that the United States had largely addressed the health care needs of the poor. Bob was among a small group who realized that the situation was more complex than this early perception, and he encouraged some of my fellow students and me to analyze the situation more closely. Some of Bob's former students, who were spread all over the country, and some of my contemporaries at Purdue and I chose to examine the use of medical services *relative* to the need for services. Both my masters thesis and doctoral dissertation examined this "need-use ratio" and how it differed for low-income black and white individuals. It was an intriguing field of investigation and enabled me to study a very important social justice issue.

When I moved to the Roanoke Valley (Virginia) in 1975—having accepted a position at Roanoke College—I discovered that a free health clinic was just in the process of getting established. I had never lived in a community with a free clinic, and I was fascinated by what it was and how it worked. I telephoned Estelle Nichols Avner, the director of the clinic, and asked if I could come down to chat with her in order to learn more. She said that she would be glad to talk to me as long as I did some work while I was there. So, while helping to move the pharmacy from one room to another in the old house being used by the clinic, I talked with Estelle and learned of the clinic's mission to offer free care to people who could not afford private care or who were otherwise disaffiliated from the private care system. She emphasized that the clinic relied on both professional and lay volunteers and that an essential part of the clinic's mission was to offer care in a relaxed, supportive, and compassionate manner.

I became a clinic volunteer, later served on the board of directors, and developed a research interest. I read available case studies of clinics, but I was surprised to find that little systematic research had been conducted. David Smith and the folks at the Haight-Ashbury Free Clinic in San Francisco had published a book, *The Free Clinic: A Community Approach to Health Care and Drug Abuse*, in 1971, and the *Journal of Social Issues* had devoted an entire issue to free clinics in 1974. Both were very helpful, but I determined that sociological analysis of free clinics and the "free clinic movement" was needed. I began with a case study of the Roanoke clinic, interviewing staff members, volunteers, and patients, and followed that with a comparative analysis of the four free clinics that existed in Virginia at that time. Later, I conducted research on the twenty existing free clinics in the southeastern part of the country and compared them with ten free clinics that had been forced to close. In each case I conducted lengthy personal interviews with the executive directors of the clinics and with other key personnel.

The idea of writing a book on free clinics crossed my mind, but I was not professionally at a point when that seemed feasible. My research interests turned to other areas, and I assumed that someone else would write what I considered to be a very important book that would tell an important story. Years later, at the turn of the century, the book had still not been written, and I committed to doing it. By this time, the story was larger and more complicated. Most of the free clinics that had emerged in the late 1960s and early 1970s had closed, while an even larger number had opened. The total number of free clinics had crept up only very slowly in the 1970s and early 1980s but had begun to increase rapidly in the late 1980s and 1990s. While almost all of the early clinics were located in large cities, many of the later clinics grew in medium-sized and smaller communities and became especially popular in the southeastern and midwestern parts of the country. These clinics had much in common with the early free clinics, but they also differed in some important respects. One of the main objectives of this book is to document and describe these important historical transformations.

I made three especially important decisions as I started on the research for this book. First, I wanted to collect as much information as possible through on-site, personal interviews. I wanted to visit free clinics, be around during clinic hours, get a feel for clinic ambience, and to see the interaction among staff, volunteers, and patients. I wanted to interview executive directors at the clinics, and when the timing and opportunity permitted, to interview other staff members and volunteers. In the beginning, I also anticipated interviewing free clinic patients, but after doing so at several clinics, I decided not to continue that aspect of the research. The patients at the clinics were sick and sometimes very sick, most did not really feel like talking, and it seemed inappropriate to ask them to sit for an interview, however brief. Instead, I determined to learn about patients from the staff and volunteers who worked with them. There are several "patient stories" included in the book, and they are compelling illustrations of patients and clinics. In order not to reveal patient identities, neither patient names, nor the clinic where services were received, nor the location of the clinic is provided for patient stories. If the story has been previously published, appropriate citations are given but not patient names.

Second, I determined that I needed to interview in clinics spread around the country. Because no one (even today) has a complete list of all free clinics, and because free clinics are continuing to be created at a rapid pace, I concluded that I should interview in various regions of the country and to base the number of interviews I conducted in an area with available information on the total number of clinics in the area (that is, doing more interviews in states like California, Virginia, and North Carolina where there are the most free clinics). Also, I wanted to interview in a cross-section of clinics: in large, medium, and small free clinics, some that had been around since the early days and some that had started in the 1980s and 1990s, some that considered themselves church-based and some that did not, and some located in large cities and some in smaller cities. There was no way to determine the quality or effectiveness of the clinic in advance, nor would I have wanted to try to do this.

The clinics in which I interviewed represent a genuine cross-section of clinics, but they were not selected strictly by a probability sampling procedure. Over about a two-year period, I visited more than forty clinics located in ten different states and the District of Columbia, conducted more than one hundred personal interviews (counting the patients interviewed), and added telephone interviews with five individuals who are prominent in the free clinic movement but whose locations I was not able to visit personally. All of the clinics contacted agreed to participate, and interviews were conducted in all but one contacted clinic—a situation where schedule conflicts made a personal interview impossible. I wish I could say that, by the end of the interviews, I had heard everything and that I would not have learned anything more from additional interviews. However, I continued to learn throughout the interview process and expect that I would have continued to learn even more if I had done additional interviews.

Finally, as much as possible, I decided to let the story of free health clinics be told by the staff and volunteers who are on the front lines. The book is filled with direct comments from my respondents. Often, the specific words and expressions that they used to answer questions are as revealing as the basic content of their replies. I saw my responsibility as doing the necessary background work, investing the time and energy in travelling to the clinics, observing and getting a feel for the clinics, formulating and asking important questions, seeking elaboration on particular answers, organizing the interviews, identifying and analyzing patterns in responses, and writing the book. In part, I hope just to stay out of the way of letting people who are passionate about their work and passionate about working with free clinic patients tell their story.

Today, there are more than 800 free health clinics in the United States. They provide health care to an estimated 3.5 million of the nation's uninsured and underinsured, they do so with tens of thousands of professional and lay volunteers, and they provide annually an estimated $3 billion in health care services. The emergence, evolution, meaning, and contributions of free health clinics represent an amazing story. It is time that it be told. I extend my deepest appreciation to all of those who shared this story with me.

I would also like to express my appreciation to all of those at Rowman & Littlefield who have contributed to this book: Alan McClare, executive editor for sociology and education; Matt Hammon, acquisitions editor for sociology and education; Alden Perkins, production editor; Jenn Nemec, associate production editor; and Stephen Beitel, copyeditor, for all of their support and assistance.

1

An Introduction to
America's Free Health Clinics

If you have seen one free health clinic . . . you have seen one free health clinic.

The free health clinic patient story that always comes to my mind is the woman in her early fifties who was brought in by her fifteen- or sixteen-year-old daughter, who wheeled her in a wheelchair. Her husband waited in the waiting room while her daughter brought her in. We asked her if she could get up on the examining table. She said that she couldn't, that she couldn't stand. We asked her if she had seen a doctor recently, and she said that she had not seen a doctor in many years. She expressed concern that her husband was working two jobs to try to make ends meet but that they had no health insurance, and she was so afraid of finding something wrong because her family could not sustain her having an illness. She reported that over the last several months, she had become weaker and was basically unable to stand. She couldn't give me any more localized symptoms than that. I took a lengthy history that was largely negative. Because she could not get up on the examination table, I proceeded to examine her [in the wheelchair]. I put my stethoscope on her chest, and she unbuttoned her blouse, and there was this devastating breast cancer that had eaten through her chest wall. I was so taken aback, because she was so clearly in denial. Her daughter was not in the room at that point, but even still, she couldn't disclose it. It was one of the most powerful patient interactions that I have ever had in my life to sit there with her and to have her explain why she couldn't be sick—that her husband couldn't know and her daughter couldn't know. There was really nothing that I could do. She was clearly dying. We sent her for an x-ray; her bones in the chest wall were just riddled with tumor. For me it identified for the first time what a healer really is. There was nothing as an organization that we could do, but I gave her an opportunity to talk. I was able to ensure her that we would be able to help with her pain, if nothing else, and that we could direct her to a facility to get her the consultation that she needed.

1

The story of America's free health clinics is as largely untold as it is revealing about clinic staff, volunteers, and patients and about the health care system. While the patient story that opens this chapter is one that is especially dramatic, each day the nation's more than 800 free health clinics quietly provide needed medical care for some of the millions of people who fall between the cracks of the medical care system safety net. Free clinics do not exist now in every community, and the resources of the existing free clinics are not adequate even to serve all of those who routinely go without needed medical care in their own communities. But, by almost any measure, free clinics offer an astounding array of medical, dental, nursing, and pharmaceutical services that are often supplemented by a host of other types of health-related and social services. These services are provided largely by professional and lay volunteers and are funded mostly through financial and in-kind contributions from individual donors and supportive groups and organizations. They are community grassroots efforts made possible by those who give their time, talents, and money to provide medical care to those who would otherwise be unable to obtain it.

A common adage among free health clinic staff and volunteers is that "if you have seen one free health clinic . . . you have seen one free health clinic." In other words, despite the presence of certain traits in most free clinics and the presence of some important general patterns, no two free clinics are exactly alike. Because free health clinics exist in all kinds of communities—with different populations who have different health problems, with a greater or lesser number of physicians and other health care professionals willing to participate, with more or less access to funding sources, and with staffs and volunteers with a wide range of personality types, leadership styles, and visions for the clinic—each free clinic is configured somewhat differently. As described later in the book, these differences represent both a significant strength of free clinics and a reason that collective organization has been complicated.

COMMON TRAITS OF FREE HEALTH CLINICS

While acknowledging these differences, a review of the organizational features of free clinics around the country suggests six important and mostly universal traits that define the core of the free clinic: free clinics (1) are community-based; (2) are private and nonprofit; (3) are volunteer-driven; (4) offer services for free or token payment; (5) emphasize compassionate care in which treating each patient with dignity is very important; and (6) focus on target populations considered most at risk within that community. This initial chapter delves into the meaning of each of these traits.

Community-Based

The fact that free health clinics are community-based means at least four specific things: (1) they are created from within communities rather than from outside agents; (2) ultimate responsibility for clinic decision making is held by individuals within the community; (3) the clinic receives funding primarily from community sources; and (4) the community takes pride in having the free clinic.

Community-Started

First, free clinics are born out of the drive and energy of one or more individuals or groups within the community. For example, the Saint Joseph Health Center in South Bend, Indiana, began with a dream of Sister (of the Holy Cross) Maura Brannick to provide free medical services to the medically unserved on the near west side of the town. Sister Brannick lived in the area, worked with the people, and had done health screenings at local soup kitchens and other facilities. With a grant from a local couple and the support of the local hospital, Saint Joseph Regional Medical Center, the clinic first opened in 1986 in a run-down old carriage house with two volunteer physicians and several volunteer nurses. In the intervening years, the clinic has twice moved to newer and larger facilities, now offers a broad range of services, and has more than 150 physician volunteers who work at the clinic or accept referrals in their offices.

The CommunityHealth Free Clinic in downtown Chicago developed from the vision of Dr. Serafino Garella, who had worked for thirty years in combating kidney disease and who was chairman of the Department of Medicine at St. Joseph Hospital on Chicago's north side. In 1991, Dr. Garella's concern was increasingly focusing on the medically uninsured. He and several of his colleagues canvassed several Chicago neighborhoods to inquire about people's health situation. They found that 40 percent of the people with whom they talked had no health insurance and were unable to get medical care. Two years of planning led in 1993 to the opening of CommunityHealth. Housed in a small storefront building and relying on volunteers, the clinic offered basic health care services at no charge to patients who walked in during the two clinic sessions each week. Quickly, it became obvious that the need was huge, and so the clinic has expanded several times in the succeeding years. Today, the clinic operates out of a large $1.3 million facility, is open six days a week, provides a broad range of medical services, and sees more than 20,000 patients each year (Cutler 2001).

The creation of the Community Clinic of High Point (North Carolina), which began seeing patients in 1993, emerged from a community needs assessment jointly conducted by the city of High Point and the local United

Way. In the assessment, health care was identified as one of four primary un-met community needs. A decision was made to begin offering care for low birth weight babies. Soon, it was suggested that the clinic also take care of the parents, and that led to a broader focus on the medically indigent. The community became more involved with support from the local urban min-istry, the Rotary Club, the Junior League, area churches, area hospitals, and from two North Carolina foundations: the Kate B. Reynolds Foundation and the Duke Endowment Fund. The clinic now provides more than 2,000 pa-tient visits each year.

In 1994, a group of physicians and nurses in the emergency room at Howard County General Hospital, the only hospital in the county in which Columbia, Maryland, is located, observed the large number of patients who had underlying illnesses such as heart disease, cancer, high blood pressure, and asthma. Some of the patients with advanced diabetes had never received medical care for it, and by the time they had come to the emergency room, they were at the point of needing amputation of their toes. These providers recognized that if these patients were receiving treatment for these chronic conditions, they would not have to make use of the more expensive and less appropriate services in the emergency room. At first, their hope was to get every physician in the area to take one additional, no-charge patient into her or his office. Soon, they decided that having a clinic would be preferable. The hospital contributed as did the local health department, individuals in the community, the county Horizon Foundation (which had been created to serve health and welfare needs), and Johns Hopkins University (which has refurbished and donated space for the clinic in a building that it owns). Thousands of patients now benefit each year at the Health Alliance for Pa-tients in Need Clinic.

In one free clinic after another, an initial vision came either from one or more individuals (often a physician but sometimes people outside medi-cine); from a church; from a social service organization; or as an outgrowth of a community needs assessment. Routinely, free clinics start with very few resources but build gradually over time into much more elaborated net-works. The Kansas City (Missouri) Free Health Clinic started in 1971 in rented rooms in an old, downtown hotel (with curtains made of tie-dyed ma-terial). The local health department donated certain necessary materials. An Episcopal church took the organizing lead; the mayor, other churches, and dental students from the University of Missouri at Kansas City, chipped in; and the clinic took root. Today, the clinic has an annual budget of more than $5.5 million, has purchased and refurbished a 23,000-square-foot facility, and provides care for more than 12,000 people each year.

The Health Care Network, Inc. Clinic in Racine, Wisconsin, grew out of community concern in the early 1980s about the number of industries that were leaving town. Lack of health care insurance for local residents was identified as a chief problem, and a specially created group, Racine 2000, energized by the tenacity of Sister Brenda Walsh of the Dominican Sisters, got the free clinic up and running in a church basement on just $25,000. Today, the clinic's budget is more than $400,000 per year, more than 200 physicians and more than forty dentists volunteer for the clinic, and more than 800 patient appointments are offered each month.

The Rockbridge (Virginia) Area Free Clinic was founded in 1991 by a local physician and insurance agent who saw the need for a grassroots effort to provide care for those who were going without needed medical services. They agreed to lead a grassroots effort to start such a facility. They attracted the support of key individuals within the community, convinced the city to donate a building for the clinic, and obtained seed money from Trigon (the name then in that area of Blue Cross–Blue Shield). They advertised for volunteers to help prepare the building, and a host of painters, interior decorators, and faculty and staff from Washington and Lee University showed up to provide the needed labor. For three years, the clinic provided care for patients without any paid staff members. Today, the annual budget for the clinic exceeds $300,000, and patients are offered general acute and chronic care, dental services, basic health examinations, women's health care, health education, and pharmaceuticals.

While every free clinic has its own origination story, there is a very common path: starting on a shoestring budget, inspired by one or two key individuals or a community group, and growing over time to try to meet widespread health care needs within the community. Importantly, the impetus for the clinics has always come from within the community itself.

Community-Directed

Second, authority and decision making for free clinics rest in the hands of individuals within the community. Almost all of the nation's free health clinics have a community-based board of directors who have ultimate responsibility for clinic policy and financial stability. Free clinics recognize that they are not all alike, and they see this as being a consequence of their freedom to tailor the clinic to the most serious health care needs within the community. It is also an outgrowth of differences in communities and in the level of access to financial support. Traditionally, free clinics have had pride in the fact that they do not rely on money from outside the community, that they are not government agencies with the attendant set of regulations, and that they do have the freedom to offer medical care in the type of atmosphere that they choose.

James Beckner, executive director of the Fan Free Clinic in Richmond, Virginia, describes his clinic in these words:

> We are the safety net. For many folks, we are the last resort. We serve the folks who don't fit in anyplace else. For instance, if you are truly indigent, you can get care. It is not going to be easy, it may not be wonderful, it can be a very difficult process, but you can access care. But if you fall into the category of working poor, you don't get care unless you are willing and able to pay out-of-pocket. Many people put themselves into financial hock for years. When we identify ourselves as the safety net below the safety net, we are a community resource. We come from the community, and we are responsible to the community. Everything here was made possible or given to us by the community. We are truly a community-based organization. Many organizations call themselves community-based, but they are taken from a model that is developed someplace else and put into and onto the community as opposed to this clinic that grew out of this community and is responsible to it.

The fact that the ultimate authority for most free clinics resides within the clinic means that clinic staff and volunteers are able to respond flexibly to unusual circumstances and not to feel constrained by outside regulations.

> We are willing to see here people who have had Medicaid and should still have Medicaid, but something has messed up with the paperwork. Nothing has changed in their status. They should still have Medicaid, but for some reason it did not recertify. We have seen cases in which even a provider who has seen them for the last five years will not see them or renew their medication. I don't understand this. Even knowing they are going to get their Medicaid again, pharmacies won't fill their medicine—they say they just can't help at all. So we see those patients here. That is the kind of thing that I don't want us ever to lose. I think we know who is falling between the cracks and what safety net needs to be out there, and we never want to be so part of the system that we lose that. (Randi Abramson, MD, Executive Director, Bread for the City/Zacchaeus Free Clinic, Washington, DC)

As an example, one of the free clinics reported the following case and its ability to do what was right regardless of its own protocols.

> A fifty-four-year-old, unemployed woman had lived in and out of dumpsters for ten years. She [had] finally accessed an organization for assistance—only it was too late. She had third-stage lung cancer and was given three to six months to live. She didn't live even the three months. However, it could be said that she died unashamedly. Had the clinic strictly defined its primary care mission, it would have sent this woman on her way, justifiably telling her: "We don't deal in temporary housing, clothing for the needy, or sponsor food programs. We don't personally engage in catastrophic care, hence, we don't do chemotherapy, we don't provide any controlled substances for any condition, we don't provide

any in-the-home visiting nurse services, and so forth, and so forth." Still, this woman—despite her grave condition—only asked for one thing: She didn't want to die in the streets, and if her fondest wish were met, she would be buried alongside her mother.

Well, despite the fact that she met our 185 percent economic criteria (standard for poverty), she really didn't "fit" into any existing program nor would it [have been] advisable to develop an arm of the clinic that would treat cancer. Still— thanks to Canton Community Clinic—all of her needs were met. As her advocate, we presented her case to those who did have such services.

She was taken into the temporary housing program at the YWCA; participated in various downtown meals programs; got some clean clothing from a local church; was included in the Stark County Visiting Nurse program—but without any charge; received all the medicines and treatments she needed to make herself comfortable—at no charge; had her affairs organized and executed by the Stark County Public Defender's Office; and she was buried beside her mother. More importantly, she didn't die in a state of pain and neglect; didn't die in a dumpster; and didn't die alone and friendless—all because she didn't fit into the mission statement of some organization. All of these services were provided at no cost through our clinic. (Canton Community Clinic 2001)

Community-Funded

Third, free clinics have been funded primarily by community dollars. This has been important for several reasons. It has given the community a sense of "symbolic ownership" of the clinic with the recognition that it would not exist except for community efforts. Community fund-raising techniques have necessarily brought the plight of the medically unserved and underserved and the need for the clinic to public attention. Many free clinics have undergone a comprehensive review process in order to qualify for United Way support. Executive directors and other staff and volunteers routinely speak to civic groups, church groups, and others to highlight the need for the clinic and the need for community dollars. And, importantly, it has enabled free clinics to avoid extending any decision-making control to external bodies and to avoid the realm of regulatory paperwork that typically accompanies external funding. This means that staff and volunteers have been free to focus on patient care.

Community dollars come from a variety of sources: local governments, United Way, financial and in-kind gifts from businesses and civic groups, church groups, local foundations, and private donations. Like many nonprofit organizations, free health clinics constantly search for creative local fund-raising projects. For example, the Rockbridge Area Free Clinic in Lexington, Virginia, benefits from an annual golf tournament and concert sponsored by NASCAR driver Rick Mast. The Los Angeles Free Clinic has benefited from fund-raising concerts by various musical artists. The Academy of

Medicine in Roanoke, Virginia, hosts an annual black-tie gala with all proceeds given to the free clinic. The Canton (Ohio) Community Clinic annually raises funds from an antique car show and auction, a pro-am golf tournament, and a night at which the local minor-league baseball team gives all ticket revenues to the clinic.

One of the most important types of community contributions is in-kind contributions provided by local hospitals and private medical laboratories. Though some free clinics receive more support from local hospitals than do other clinics, the vast majority of free clinics receive certain services (such as radiology services) from hospitals at no charge or at greatly reduced charge. In some communities private medical laboratories donate some services to the free clinic as a community contribution.

Of the four components of being community-based, this is the only one that has changed significantly over time as an increasing number of clinics now obtain some financial support from state and local grant programs (in a few cases, from federal grant programs) and from foundations outside the community. West Coast clinics are more likely than clinics elsewhere to secure contracts with government bodies to provide designated services. This has been a significant step for these free clinics and one that has sometimes been controversial. But the need for services is so great that clinics have looked to new areas for financial support.

Community-Supported

Finally, being community-based suggests a type of community pride in having the free clinic. Logically, this pride is more evident in smaller communities that have only a single free clinic and that receive the focus of the entire community. Ironically, free clinics located in communities with only one hospital often receive more in-kind support from that single hospital than clinics located in communities with more than one hospital receive from the hospitals collectively. This pattern is consistent with a "diffusion of responsibility" interpretation: when there is only one hospital, responsibility for assisting the clinic clearly falls to that hospital, and the necessary support will not be available unless that hospital provides it. In multihospital communities, it is easier for each hospital to step back, hoping that one of the others provides the needed support. In addition, in the very competitive world of medical organizations, hospitals in multihospital communities often want to and do contribute to important local causes but, at the same time, are resentful if the entire burden of support falls only on them. Nevertheless, there is evident community pride that is enjoyed by free clinics around the country, and the free clinics appreciate this feeling and recognize its importance.

Beyond the typical indicators of community support, many of the clinics that are located within or adjacent to residential neighborhoods have received special benefits from residents of the neighborhood. Some of the clinics are located in high-crime areas, and they often receive special protection from neighbors or neighborhood watch groups. Recently, when a young man broke a window in a South Carolina clinic, an elderly woman across the street, who observed the incident, promptly nabbed him and made him clean up the mess. For a time, a motorcycle gang lived in a house next door to an Indiana clinic. The neighborhood was not always a safe place, but members of the gang served as unofficial protectors of the clinic and ensured that there were never any problems there. An Ohio clinic director said this about the clinic's neighbors:

We are located in a pretty rough neighborhood which is why we are not open in evenings and at night. But the kids are always willing to come over and cut the grass when it gets long. I have been told that the clinic and everything associated with the clinic is off-limits to gangs. It is a designated, protected area. The neighborhood appreciates and respects what the clinic does. (Eric Riley, Executive Director, Canton Community Clinic, Canton, Ohio)

David Smith, founder and director of the Haight-Ashbury Free Clinics, which have significant identification with that section of the city, says it this way:

Community involvement is an essential component of the clinic. The community views the clinic as an integral service; we have a broad-based board of directors; and we deliver a service that the community needs. We are firmly rooted in the community, we patronize the businesses, and we contribute to the overall health of Haight-Ashbury. We have a strong base of community support, and we do not want to be perceived as an outside institution.

Whoever took the first step and however it was taken, a hallmark of free clinics is that they gain widespread community support in terms of financial and in-kind contributions, volunteers, public recognition, and neighborhood support.

Private and Nonprofit

Most free health clinics are recognized by the Internal Revenue Service as 501(c)(3) agencies. This is the typical designation in the United States for nonprofit organizations including those that are primarily civic, religious, or public service–oriented. To qualify, an organization must be focused on public service rather than on making money. The primary benefits of 501(c)(3) status are an exemption from paying taxes, the ability of donors to receive a tax deduction for contributions to the organization, eligibility to receive public and private grant funds and to participate in select government programs, and limited liability for members of the board of directors, employees, and volunteers.

In addition, free clinics typically are private rather than public (government-sponsored) organizations. They are answerable to a board of directors rather than being part of a federal, state, or local government agency, although they can and many do receive funds from government bodies. The board of directors in some free clinics is comprised primarily of members of the health care professions—in some cases, drawn heavily from their own volunteers—while other boards represent a broader cross-section of the community. Boards are ultimately responsible for the policy making and fiscal integrity of the clinic.

Free clinics cover a wide spectrum from, on the one hand, being completely secular organizations to, on the other hand, being faith-based. But the relationship is even more complicated than that. Even most of the secular clinics receive some support from churches and have some staff and volunteers who are motivated out of a spiritually or religiously based desire to contribute to others. And, conversely, the more openly faith-based clinics have staff and volunteers who are not religious and whose motivations for being at the clinic have a more secular, humanitarian basis. Only one clinic in which I interviewed conceived of the clinic as a means to recruit parishioners. Rather, the clinics that are faith-based view that in terms of service and are intentionally welcoming of all interested staff and volunteers, whatever their spiritual or religious beliefs.

The configuration of funding for free clinics is based largely on the ability and willingness to donate by individuals and organizations within the community. Financial support from corporations, foundations, and the local or state government is also typical. Because communities are so different, a wide diversity of funding arrangements exists.

For example, in West Virginia, the Division of Primary Care of the State Health Department allots money to primary care clinics, and free clinics receive allocations from this allotment. This sum, which represents as much as half or more of the budget in some free clinics, is then supplemented by various forms of community funding.

In Virginia, private donations typically are one of the largest sources of funding, but donations from private and civic organizations, the United Way, churches, government grants for particular programs (e.g., diabetes programs or dental care programs), and annual fund-raisers are all common. The state legislature now allocates more than a million dollars annually to the Virginia Association of Free Clinics, which in turn allocates funds to the almost fifty free clinics in the state.

Free clinics that are located in the largest metropolitan areas typically face the most pressure to expand fund-raising beyond private gifts. The CommunityHealth Clinic in Chicago, one of the nation's largest clinics, solicits no government grants or reimbursements but uses funds from private foundations to cover almost two-thirds of its $1 million annual budget. An annual benefit brings in another 25 percent of funds, while voluntary patient donations have accounted for more than $30,000 annually in recent years.

Expansion of fund-raising to sources outside the community—especially acceptance of government grants—creates a complex issue for free clinics. The desire to avoid significant bureaucratic elements and excessive regulation must be tempered with the need to monitor programs and to document compliance with funders' requirements. The desire to be free to move the clinic as patient needs dictate must be reconciled with the importance of raising as much money as possible to address those patient needs. The movement of some free clinics toward contracts with local, state, and federal governments is discussed in more detail in chapter 9.

Volunteer-Driven

A key component of free health clinics is a reliance on health care professional and lay volunteers to staff the clinic. As the size of individual clinics has grown, as services have expanded, as paperwork requirements have increased, and as the number of patients seen has grown and grown, the number of full-time and part-time paid staff positions also has increased. However, the typical free clinic model continues to be an organization with a small number of paid staff and a very large number of volunteers. This is part of the community foundation of free clinics and part of what makes them grassroots organizations.

For example, the Venice Family Clinic in Venice, California, may be the nation's largest free health clinic. For its first seven years of existence, it was an entirely volunteer-run clinic offering services out of a dental office. Then, over a period of years, the clinic leased a small medical office, moved to a new building (with 30,000 patient contacts per year), renovated and enlarged the building (moving to 50,000 patient contacts per year), and in the mid-1990s, assumed control of two county clinics that were about to close. The clinic now provides 90,000 patient contacts per year to around 18,000 patients. This is accomplished with only twelve paid positions but with more than 2,000 volunteers of whom about 500 are physicians. Together they offer a wide range of services including prenatal, pediatric, adult episodic and preventive, diabetes, hypertension, asthma, heart disease, women's health care (well-woman and breast and cervical cancer screening), along with a full range of specialist care, an HIV program, health education, and mental health counseling.

The DuPage Community Clinic in Wheaton, Illinois, has a $500,000 annual budget and provides approximately 11,000 patient visits per year. While there are several paid staff members, all of the physicians are volunteers. As

at most free health clinics, some volunteer physicians come in evenings after working the entire day, while others give up part of their day off to work
at the clinic. Others accept clinic-referred patients at no charge in their private office. The clinic is open to see patients from 8:00 a.m. to 4:00 p.m. on
weekdays (the nurse practitioner–medical director is always available during
these hours) and, on one evening each week, the clinic remains open until
9:00 p.m. and is staffed by volunteer physicians. Among the many services
offered are those for general acute care, diabetes, hypertension, ADHD,
women's health (pap smears and mammograms), and dental services.

The Davidson Medical Ministries Clinic in Lexington, North Carolina, is located in a small town of about 14,000 people and is surrounded by a county
with a population of about ten times that number. With an annual budget of
more than $500,000, the clinic provides about $2 million in annual care. Last
year, almost 200 volunteers provided more than 12,000 volunteer hours to
help staff the clinic. Davidson schedules clinics both to maximize use of volunteer health care professionals and to be available when needed by patients.

> The medical clinic is open on Monday and Thursday evening. Patients make ap-
> pointments at 2:00 in the afternoon on a first-come, first-served basis. We have
> a small pool of key providers; if we do not have a provider that evening, we will
> not have clinic. For the clinic, we use volunteer doctors, dentists, nurses, phar-
> macists, front desk receptionists, social workers, eligibility screening lay volun-
> teers, medical/dental/pharmacy support staff, and full-time staff supervisors.
> Tuesday morning is medicine refill pick-up day. Tuesday afternoon is the nurs-
> ing clinic—nursing students come in and see patients who need follow-up, they
> do lab work, they do teaching, they provide tender loving care, and they do
> home visits for those who cannot get to the clinic if they need a blood pressure
> check or if the clinic thinks it would benefit from knowing what the living con-
> dition is like. Also, a chronic disease clinic focusing on diabetes and hyperten-
> sion operates on Tuesday afternoon; it is funded by a grant from the Duke En-
> dowment Fund for a part-time physician assistant and a grant from the Kate B.
> Reynolds Foundation for diabetes case management. This is a comprehensive
> managed care clinic for patients who are pulled out of our general medical clin-
> ics on Monday and Thursday.
>
> A pharmacist is here on Wednesday morning to provide medications for
> Medicare patients. They are asked to show up every month on the same
> Wednesday. Wednesday is also a chronic disease clinic and nursing clinic and
> eligibility screening. Thursday is another medication refill day. We have a part-
> nership with the health department for a children's Medicaid dental clinic; the
> health department does not have a dental facility so the DMS facility is used. We
> are open 42 hours per week. If each clinic operated independently, we would
> be providing 150 hours of service per week. Typically, the medical clinic is open
> from 6:00 to 9:00 p.m. Monday and Thursday, but some providers prefer an ear-
> lier or later start. Appointment hours are matched to provider availability and
> preferences. (Sandy Motley, Executive Director, Davidson Medical Ministries
> Clinic, Inc., Lexington, North Carolina)

In addition to enhancing community identification with the clinic, the extensive use of volunteers has important financial and fund-raising implications. Typically, free clinics are able to leverage the dollars donated into three or four or more times their actual value. The net value of the volunteer help is in the thousands or hundreds of thousands of dollars at most clinics and is valued at more than a million dollars at a few of the largest clinics. So, for example, a contribution to a free clinic that enables hiring a staff member who, in turn, recruits volunteers or solicits in-kind contributions extends the total value of services provided by much more than its face amount.

> In all of my research, free clinics are the one charity in the United States that can take one dollar and turn it into five or six. I remember one article in *United States News and World Report* or *Money Magazine* that said, on average, of each charitable dollar given, seventy-five cents actually goes to the charity. Free clinics are one place where a dollar can be turned into several times the given amount. (Tom Rives, MD, a long-standing contributor to the Friendship House Free Clinic in Conway, South Carolina)

This can also be an effective fund-raising appeal, and many clinics have carefully calculated the "bang for the buck" of contributions that they receive. With increasing societal concern that donations to charitable groups end up paying for administrative costs and future fund-raising appeals, the knowledge that contributions to free clinics have "extra" value can be a persuasive technique.

Services Offered for Free or Token Payment

Most free health clinics provide their services at no charge whatsoever to patients. Some ask for or mention the option of a very modest donation (where this occurs, it may be one or two dollars per patient), and some clinics now request a specific but very low fee for services that are very expensive for the clinic to provide. While many government-sponsored medical clinics operate on a sliding-scale basis (that is, the fee is proportionate to income so that those with less income pay smaller fees), free clinics do not follow this model. Some prefer a token fee arrangement with the rationale that patients who contribute something to the cost will feel better about themselves and be more invested in following treatment regimens, but the vast majority of free clinics do not charge any fees.

All free clinics have had to make some determination about whether or not to have eligibility requirements or to have patients undergo any type of means test to qualify to be seen at the free clinic. Many clinics are opposed in principle to having eligibility requirements. For example, the Fan Free Clinic in Richmond, Virginia, collects some financial information from patients but does not use it to screen for eligibility. Services are available to anyone who requests them as long as there is space and staff to help them. The Free Clinic of Greater Cleveland in Ohio follows the same protocol. However, both clinics work to connect their patients with other social services in the community that are needed, and some patients may be counseled to use other available services. But these and some other clinics do not want to discourage anyone from coming to the clinic for fear they would not be eligible to be seen.

Sairah Husain, coordinator of the Information and Referral Collective at the Berkeley Free Clinic, describes this orientation in her clinic:

> We do not require identification for any of our services because that makes it a lot easier for some people to come in. Anyone can come in. We want people to come even if they have insurance. We don't ask if you have insurance; we don't bill insurance; we want to see people if they want to be seen.

Clinics that use eligibility requirements justify them on one or the other or both of two grounds. First, the clinic wants to make its services maximally available to people who genuinely need the services and would not have access to any services if not for the free clinic. No clinic has too much money. Therefore, if a patient has the means to be seen elsewhere, and is counseled to do so, it would mean greater availability for those without service options. Second, because free clinics rely on volunteers, they want to ensure that only patients who cannot afford private care are seen at the clinic. The concern is that motivation to volunteer, especially by health care professionals, would diminish if they were giving their time and being asked to treat patients who do not really need free clinic services.

Clinics that do screen for eligibility typically try to do so in a nonintrusive manner. They focus on income relative to the federally established poverty level and do not see patients who have private health insurance, Medicare, or Medicaid. In some clinics, patients may qualify only if they have no insurance and earn less than 100 percent of the federally established poverty level. Other clinics use a different percentage, which may range between 100 percent up to more than 200 percent. Most are careful to retain some flexibility for special cases—and free clinics see many special cases.

For example, in Joliet, Illinois, eligibility to use the Will-Grundy Medical Center was set at 180 percent of the poverty level and no insurance. However, members of the board of directors conducted a systematic inquiry into area costs for rent, food, and other essentials. They determined that it would be very difficult to afford private medical care for individuals and families earning up to 220 percent of the poverty level. Eligibility was revised to the 220 percent level.

Patients who can make a donation often do so, either in cash or in-kind. Marilynn Bridges, the executive director of the Free Clinic of Franklin County in Rocky Mount, Virginia, and Karon Jones, clinical services director of the clinic, can easily recount various gifts that patients have made or grown and brought to them, including cakes, various kinds of produce, and crocheted slippers. Laura Michalski, director of clinical relations at CommunityHealth in Chicago also recalls patient gifts ranging from flowers to baked goods. Parker Sparrow, executive director of The Free Medical Clinic (of Columbia, South Carolina), recounted this humorous (in retrospect) example of patients giving back:

On one night, the toilet was leaking in the women's bathroom. So I go look at it and see that the leak is coming from one of the pipes under the seat. I did not want to spend the money to call a plumber, because we try to get as much donated as we can. I went out into the waiting room and asked if anybody in there was a plumber. The patients started laughing, but two guys said they knew a little bit about it, and one said that we needed some kind of bolt. The other guy said that he was not a plumber, but if we made sure to hold his place in line, he would run over to the plumbing warehouse right around the corner, and get what we needed. He did and came back and fixed it. I asked him to give me the receipt so we could repay him, but he refused and said that we already do so much for him.

Emphasis on Compassionate Care and Patient Dignity

Staff and volunteers in free health clinics across the country emphasize that the clinic is more than just a free care site. Part of the overall commitment of clinics is to emphasize the delivery of care with compassion and with respect for the dignity of the patients. It would be hard to imagine that this heightened level of respect characterizes every volunteer and staff member and every encounter between them and patients. But free clinics take this value very seriously, and it is a fundamental part of their core values.

Entering providers must understand the "culture of caring" of the clinic. This is not the place that you come when you want to walk in, quickly see a patient, treat them, and urge them out the door. It is a place where you develop a relationship that is unique with those who come to the clinic. You give them all the time that they want; you listen to them, you find out about them more than the lab data and the test material, because we don't think of them as patients or as diseases, or God forbid, anything as impersonal as a chart. We consider them as a friend or neighbor who doesn't feel well. We'll try to help them. That is so important because everything else that happens from the time they enter the clinic till they are on the way out is dictated by that one perception. And sometimes providers might come in and think they are going to give patients some pills, and then they will walk on out, and the patients will be grateful. It is the caregivers who need to be grateful because they receive every bit as much, if they allow themselves to, as the recipient. (Jack McConnell, MD, Founder, Volunteers in Medicine Clinic, Hilton Head Island, South Carolina)

It is very important that we convey a warm, loving, and compassionate attitude to our patients . . . because we feel that way. And to let them know that we care, we care about their lives. . . . (Parker Sparrow, Executive Director, The Free Medical Clinic, Columbia, South Carolina)

A good gauge of the people coming through the door is something that Father Alfred (Bodecur, the founder of the clinic) insisted upon in all of our services— an environment that is rooted in dignity and respect. That has been our foundation in all of our work. And, I think, especially when you look at the conditions in which many of our folks live, in all of our services, the barometer for us is that as people are received in dignity, they in turn reflect that back. (Thomas Gleason, Director of Development and Communications, St. Anthony Free Medical Clinic, San Francisco, California)

People can tell if you care or you don't. It makes a difference when people know that you care, that you are doing what you can. They still have to do their part, but our patients respond to that because in many cases, people have never really expressed care for them. They have been labeled, they have been stereotyped. They are so used to the system turning its back on them . . . some of them are very angry, and it takes a while to establish rapport. (Judy Dillow, Director of the First Baptist Church of North Charleston [South Carolina] Clinic)

Several of the respondents who were interviewed for this book could recount at least one occasion when, at the end of a clinic session, a volunteer was thanked for his or her contribution but asked not to return on the basis that he or she had failed to offer genuinely caring and respectful interaction with patients. Staff and volunteers emphasize to patients that there is absolutely nothing to be ashamed of in obtaining medical services at a free health clinic, and that free clinic patients deserve the respect that we would like to see every patient receive in every setting. Most patients interviewed spontaneously commented on this aspect of their care. Several staff and volunteers commented on the fact that they rarely received as much courtesy or respectful treatment at their private care site as patients receive at the free clinic.

It is very important that we respect where they are and we treat them with respect because they are our fellow human beings and our neighbors. By the grace of God go any of us—that we might lose our health care. We work hard to make them comfortable and to say that this is an okay place for now, that you need to be here, and we are here to help you where life has you at the moment. (Lee Elmore, Executive Director, North Coast Health Ministry Clinic, Lakewood, Ohio)

I will share with you a story of a patient who came to the clinic several times over a period of about two years. He was a very thin African-American male who was in poor general health, although he did not have any life-threatening conditions. When he would come in, we would always just spend some time talking about his life, but he would always also ask me about my life. One time, he stayed outside until clinic was over and caught me on my way out. He was crying. He apologized for that and said he did not want other patients to see him being so emotional. He asked if he could give me a hug to thank me for caring about him. During our hug, I was also crying.

Targeted on At-Risk Groups

Because free health clinics are community organizations, they are free to focus on whatever group or groups within the community seem most at risk. Some free clinics have targeted homeless people within the community. Some have targeted those who are unable to purchase medications. Some provide extensive programs for substance abusers. However, as described in more detail in chapters 2 and 3, changing circumstances in the country and changes in the availability of other programs have led most communities today to identify the "working poor" as the group most at risk. These are individuals and families who work (often full-time), do not have health insurance, do not earn enough money to pay for private medical care, but earn "too much" money to qualify for medical assistance programs. These patients lack access to basic health care services and are the common focus for most free health clinics.

Staff and volunteers shared the following stories as illustrations:

Some of our patients work at jobs that offer health insurance, but it is so expensive that they cannot afford it. One couple with three children made $760 per month after taxes. It would cost $260 a month to pay the employee portion of health insurance for just the husband and wife. Thanks to a special program, the kids could be covered for an additional $45 total. Given all of their other expenses, paying more than $300 per month for health insurance was unaffordable.

One of our patients was a man who drove a city bus. He did not have health insurance, and he could not afford private care, so he simply stopped going to see a physician. When he came to us, he said that he had swollen ankles. We quickly examined him and found that he was in congestive heart failure. We called the rescue squad and got him to the hospital in time.

For several years, I did medical and social histories on patients when they arrived at the free clinic. In the early years, we saw many children. I would take the parent or parents and the child into the interview room and learn everything I could about the child's illness—the reason for the visit. Then, I would ask about the parents' health. And, even though they had not come to the clinic to be seen themselves, with some encouragement, they very frequently opened up and revealed medical problems they were having. I remember some occasions where they had waited too long. But usually we were able to help. Yet, what struck me the most was that these folks had simply given up on getting care for themselves. Their concern was for the children, and sometimes they had grown so weary of being turned away from private care or being treated disrespectfully, that they had simply given up. If I live to be a hundred, I will never, never forget these people and these conversations.

One of our patients was a young mother who was working at two nursing homes. Both hired her part-time so that they did not have to provide health insurance. She earned just above the minimum wage and could not afford health insurance. She had a seventeen-year-old daughter who was complaining about chest pain. The mom admitted that she had ignored the girl for a while, because she was seventeen, and kids that age are always complaining about something, so she really did not pay too much attention. But the daughter kept complaining. She took her to the emergency room two or three times, and they never found anything, so she stopped doing that. The girl kept complaining about chest pain.

Finally, she went to some of the nurses at the nursing home and asked if anything could be done and, if so, what it would be. One of these nurses told the mother about our program. She brought the girl in, and, at first, we didn't know what the problem was, but we set her up to see a doctor on-site here. The doctor examined her and came to me immediately saying that we need to get her to a surgeon stat. So we got her in right away to see a surgeon, and by the end of the week, she had a baseball-size mass taken out of her breast. When it was happening, we were all thinking about that poor kid, but the part that really struck me happened later when the mother was thanking us profusely and saying that she felt so terrible that she took care of other people's family members all day long, yet she couldn't even take care of her own daughter. My heart ached for her because this was a mother who wanted to do right for her daughter, did everything she could within her resources, and was a working mom, yet still had to go through this terrible ordeal. The daughter turned out well, but a little later, she might not have.

Free clinics also are at the forefront of dealing with the effects of the extremely high price of medications in this country. Even patients who are able to access medical care often have a difficult or impossible time paying for prescription medicines. For many patients, the cost of drugs is simply prohibitive. Not surprisingly, therefore, most free clinics have a pharmacy or dispensary and work with patients to try to help them secure needed medications. Essentially all free clinic patients require this type of assistance. Plus, even though few free clinics see Medicare patients (because Part B of Medicare pays for medical care), many will provide medications for these patients (because, until recently, Medicare did not include any prescription drug benefit).

A lady called up to see if she would be eligible to receive medications from the free clinic. Her income was $991 per month. And, so I thought goodness, we have people who are getting less than half that per month, and I wondered why she wasn't able to make do on $991 for one person. Then, she told me about her medications, and they cost $779 per month. We weren't able to provide everything that she took, but we covered three-fourths of them.

We see many couples over the age of sixty-five who have worked their entire life and, at some point, had enough money to buy a house. When we see them, they are on Medicare and Social Security. Their combined income is often less than $1,000 a month. Together, the household may be on fifteen to twenty medications for diabetes, hypertension, arthritis, etc. Their drug costs per month exceed their entire income.

2

The Emergence
of Free Health Clinics

They came out of the 1960s like marshals taming the West, determined to
make medical care more available and more dignified. . . .

William Doll, 1985

THE SOCIAL AND CULTURAL BACKGROUND

The 1960s was one of those decades that occurs two or three times a century
and has a profound transformative effect on society. It was a decade that spilled
over into the seventies and whose effects are still rippling through some of our
more remote social bayous even as the reaction to those effects dominates the
societal center. (Freeman 1983, xiii)

The emergence of free health clinics in the 1960s was both part of the important social and cultural changes of that decade and a reaction to them. To
fully understand the milieu in which free clinics came into being, it is necessary to understand the broader social and cultural context. Clearly, reference
to the "1960s" as an entity unto itself is something of a misnomer. It is merely
a literary device to refer to a very tense and a very intense period of time in
United States history that may best be seen as starting in the mid-1950s and
ending sometime in the early 1970s during Richard Nixon's presidential administration. While the popular adage is that "if you can remember the
1960s, you must not have been a part of it," many analysts identify it as a—
if not the—pivotal time period of the second half of the twentieth century.

In a cogent analysis of the decade, John Judis (1998) contends that this
time period ought to be divided into two phases. The first phase runs from

December 1955, when Rosa Parks refused to give up her seat on a segregated Montgomery, Alabama, public bus to around 1965. This phase includes the rise of Martin Luther King, Jr., and the Southern civil rights movement; the advent of campus activism including the founding of Students for a Democratic Society (SDS); passage of several civil rights bills, Medicare, Medicaid, and the War on Poverty (which may be viewed as a belated continuation of the progressive era and Franklin D. Roosevelt's New Deal programs). Publication of Michael Harrington's *The Other America* brought to popular attention the fact that many people were not sharing in societal prosperity, and daily news reports showed the vehemence of racial prejudice and discrimination. Still, many perceive that this period of time was characterized by a general optimism. Many believed that America would be able to produce enough abundance so that those who were being left out of prosperity—the poor, the aged, and the disadvantaged—could share in the "good life" if only appropriate government programs could be created.

The second phase of this time period—running from 1965 to about 1973 or 1974—reflects a darker, less optimistic, and more violent period of American history. This period begins with the escalation of the war in Southeast Asia and the riots in American cities, and it continues through the rise of the black power and militant antiwar movements. The assassinations of Robert Kennedy and Martin Luther King, Jr., in 1968 added both to despair and outrage. In 1969 Students for a Democratic Society (SDS) broke into factions, and the most radical faction, the Weathermen, capturing media headlines for its increased willingness to lay nonviolent approaches aside.

However, seeds of other social movements, which had been planted in the earlier phase, also came to fruition during the latter phase. The women's movement brought individual and public attention to gender inequities and institutionalized gender discrimination, the environmental movement rallied those who were concerned about the continued degradation of the natural environment, attention to the rights of consumers was stimulated by the work of Ralph Nader and others, and the Gray Panthers formed to work against age discrimination.

During this second phase, college and high school students became increasingly visible participants in many of these movements. By the mid- to late-1960s, it had become increasingly common to refer to a "youth culture," "youth counterculture," or just "the counterculture," and in 1970, the presidentially appointed Commission on Campus Unrest identified the clash between youth culture and mainstream society as a threat to stability within the country.

While current analyses sometimes gloss over important differences among young people during this time, there were some very important differences. At one end of the spectrum, many college students in the sixties were, at least on the surface, relatively unchanged by and uninterested in social and political events, and they were occasionally disgusted that the world had infringed on their good times. Other students were heavily involved in social activism and were dedicated members of social movements. While some activists in the late sixties became committed to violent strategies (and received much media attention), they were never more than a small minority of young social activists, and most adhered to using nonviolent approaches to effecting change.

Rather than seeking changes in America's underlying value structure, many of these young social activists sought to challenge the country to live up to its stated ideals. Their activism often was motivated by disillusionment with politicians who failed to be candid about the conduct of the war in Southeast Asia. Their anger was directed at those who spoke of ideals yet did whatever they could to deny basic freedoms and justice to people of color, to women, and to the poor. Public efforts of these activists were designed to raise people's awareness of social issues and social problems, to force enforcement of laws already passed, and to pass additional laws aimed at guaranteeing social justice.

A third group of young people during this time can be distinguished by their rejection of mainstream society's basic values. Often referred to as "hippies" (a takeoff on Norman Mailer's "hipster"), this group followed Harvard professor Dr. Timothy Leary's advice to "tune in, turn on, and drop out."

> The so-called "hippie movement" started in major cities across the United States in the middle 1960s, and San Francisco became one of the centers of attraction for dissatisfied youth. These young persons were born in an era of affluence; they did not live through the depression or the World Wars, nor could they identify with the goal-oriented, self-righteous, mechanized way of life practiced by their parents. They were asked to participate in an armed conflict in a faraway land which they could not understand or condone. Their dress, tendency to live communally, sexual freedom, and, above all, use of drugs and reluctance to work in any steady occupation separated them from the traditional "clean-cut" American teenager.
>
> Many of these hippies were from affluent, middle- and upper-class families. They formed a new group of young people, concerned more with the existential experience of the "Here and Now" (immediate relationships and gratification) and with trying to find a meaning to their existence other than an eventual seat on the board of directors of some large company. (Galbis 1971)

The hippies frequently lived communally, and sought a spiritual existence based on peace, love, and tranquility. They were not job-obsessed or materialism-driven. They engaged in casual sex, "crashed' anyplace that was available, often failed to get enough to eat, and abused powerful drugs (increasingly LSD—a psychedelic drug that was considered to be mind-expanding). Getting "hassled" by the general public and getting "busted" by the police were constant concerns. It was an unhygienic and, in many ways, health-harming lifestyle. The need for comprehensive and continuous medical care was great.

However, establishment medicine frequently turned its back on these young people. Many physicians personally objected to the youth counterculture and allowed their own values to negatively affect their interaction with young social activists and hippies. Some medical providers believed that the lifestyle chosen by these young people justified denying them any right to medical care. When these young people sought medical attention for drug-related health problems, physicians sometimes treated them disrespectfully and condescendingly and sometimes turned them in to the local police. Even physicians who were entirely willing to treat these young people often were by and large completely untrained to deal with drug abuse and were not able to offer optimal care.

> For years the black residents of the ghetto have known what the hip white drug user is finding out—that there is a double standard for health care just as there is for criminal justice. Doctors don't like to treat hippies and street people, and especially drug users. It's not good for business. The client of the health care professional has to be socially acceptable. (Smith, Bentel, and Schwartz 1971, xi)

The mutual disrespect that developed led many young people to refuse to seek medical care. Drug users did their best to treat each other and often developed some useful knowledge, but they did so without the facilities and resources of professional medicine. It was this situation—a tremendous need for medical care that was not being met by establishment medicine—that led to the creation of the first free clinics.

> Community health care clinics, or "free clinics" as they are called, were not created as novel community experiments, demonstration projects, or even as pilot programs, nor were they the result of social dilettantism by social reformers. They emerged out of acute need and sheer desperation. They were also not part of what Selznick has called "a broad, conscious, social vision," but were established, ad hoc, to cope with an epidemic of youthful drug abuse and the health problems which accompany it. (Smith, Bentel, and Schwartz 1971, x)

THE EARLY FREE CLINICS

As many of these young people migrated to urban areas, they created significant pockets of the youth counterculture. Extensive drug-related problems, sexually transmitted and other types of infections, problem pregnancies, problems related to lack of nutrition and sanitation, and a host of other acute illnesses became common in these areas. San Francisco was an especially popular destination for young people from all over the country, and it is there that Dr. David Smith took steps to create the first free health clinic, The Haight-Ashbury Free Clinic, in June 1967. (The Haight-Ashbury Free Clinic is described in more detail later in this chapter.)

Quickly, free clinics emerged in other cities around the country. Later in 1967, free clinics emerged in Seattle, Cincinnati, and Detroit (and in Vancouver, Canada). In the following year, free clinics were started in Boston, Cambridge (MA), Philadelphia, Chicago (two), Champaign (IL), Cincinnati (two more), Minneapolis, St. Louis, the District of Columbia, Chapel Hill (NC), Durham (NC), Atlanta, Denver, Las Vegas, Pasadena, San Bernardino (CA), San Francisco (one more), Portland (OR), and Bellevue (WA) (and in Montreal and Winnipeg, Canada).

Types of Free Clinics

After just three years, it was apparent that three types of free clinics were emerging: hippie drug clinics (also called street clinics), neighborhood (minority) clinics, and youth clinics (Smith, Bentel, and Schwartz 1971). *Hippie drug clinics* focused on providing medical services—with an emphasis on drug abuse treatment—for transient young people. Services typically included detoxification and rehabilitation treatment, counseling, and care for drug-related acute illnesses. *Neighborhood (minority) clinics* were usually created by politically organized racial and ethnic minority group members to address the unmet medical needs of their group. Examples are inner-city medical clinics run by the Black Panthers and medical programs for migrant workers run by Chicanos. These clinics offered fairly comprehensive medical services to people of all ages. *Youth clinics* were usually establishment medicine–based clinics that focused on life education and drug education and counseling and were targeted at high school students (these clinics were quickly folded into other programs).

Characteristics of the Early Hippie Drug Clinics

Most of the early free clinics were hippie drug clinics. Many of the core elements of free health clinics described in chapter 1 were present in these early clinics, at least in rudimentary form. Clinics were routinely started in church basements or in buildings donated by churches or in run-down storefronts. Most (in many cases—all) of the equipment and supplies were donated. Patients were not charged any fee for medical care. There was little paperwork maintained, and no eligibility requirements. All or most of the providers were volunteers. Emphasis was placed on treating patients with respect, being nonjudgmental, and to offering care in as informal of an environment as possible: no formal medical garb, and physicians and other providers usually dressed in jeans and introduced themselves by their first name. Walls often reflected the psychedelic posters or paint common at the time. The intended message was clear: establishment medicine had largely turned its back on these patients, but this was not establishment medicine.

Sociologist and attorney William Doll (1985, 8) described these early clinics:

> Defiantly Goodwill in decor, militantly compassionate in demeanor, they came out of the 1960s like marshalls taming the West, determined to make medical care more available and more dignified. . . .
>
> For no pay and long hours, they took on the maladies and personal confusions other doctors and other clinics either couldn't or wouldn't treat.

To these early free clinic contributors, the term "free" in the name of the clinic referred to much more than the provision of services without charge. It was designed to convey that many of the discomforting features of establishment medicine were not part of free clinic medicine.

> The term free clinic means more than just no patient charge per visit. It also means no probing questions, no "morality trips," no red tape, no files, no labeling or judging, no "put downs," but an effort to run a humane service center. A person is not just labeled a "junky" or a "speed freak," but is first a person. Clinics are in great part run and operated by non-professionals without any official credentials, but working in collaboration with a few credentialed individuals. (Smith, Bentel, and Schwartz 1971, xiv)

Characteristics of the Early Neighborhood Clinics (Minority)

While the patients served in hippie drug clinics tended to be of high school and college age, white, middle-class, and estranged from their families and society, the neighborhood clinics were established primarily to serve racial and ethnic minority group members (whether African American, Latino, Native American, or Asian) of all ages whose health care needs were systematically not being met by the organized medical care system. The exclusion of these racial and ethnic minority group members from establishment medicine often was based on an inability to pay for private care, but sometimes could be traced to the shortage of available medical providers in minority communities and sometimes to the absence of respect and dignity in the way that minority patients were treated when they did access the system. As William Harvey (1974) stated in the early 1970s, it did not make any difference to these individuals what the clinic was called or what the source of its financing was; it only mattered that care was offered for free and that patients were treated with respect and compassion.

Harry Clark of the Free People's Clinic in Ann Arbor, Michigan (1974, 67–68), stated the rationale for establishing neighborhood clinics in black residential areas:

Inasmuch as the traditional vehicles of health care delivery fail to make available to the black populace adequate health care, and because the traditional health care structure has proven itself to be indifferent or overtly hostile to the health requirements of the black community, it is incumbent on the black community to react to the void created by this neglect and to deal with the basic health needs of its constituents; it is incumbent on the black community to create a milieu which is not psychologically traumatic to its people, a milieu which does not presume the lack of human dignity and encourage casual and paternalistic care, a milieu that does not presume that the lack of monetary reserve supposes an availability to substandard care or to experimentation, a milieu which does not create a white magic of health care delivery with warlocks and witches as intermediaries to the masses.

Though the target population in the hippie drug clinics and the neighborhood clinics was different, the features of the early clinics had much in common. Neighborhood clinics also tended to be in storefront or church basement locations, also relied on donated equipment and volunteers, also emphasized the importance of treating patients with respect and dignity, and also did away with as much red tape as possible. The most pronounced difference between the two types of clinics centered on the extent to which the clinics were intended to make a political statement and the extent to which staff and volunteers wanted the clinic to be in the forefront of significant social change. Many—though not all—of those in the hippie drug clinics saw the free clinic as a gateway to working for significant change in the overall health care system, so that their focus was on sociopolitical change as well as patient services. The focus for many—though not all—of those in the neighborhood minority clinics was centered more fully on patient services. In the early 1970s, staff and volunteers in these clinics interpreted the increasing number of free clinics less as a broad social movement and more as opportunities to address the basic health care needs of underserved populations.

The Struggles of the Early Free Clinics

For most of the early free clinics, just staying open was a major preoccupation. While they often were successful in getting a site and secondhand equipment donated, money was required to sustain clinic operations, and money was often in short supply. Clinic volunteers invested considerable time and effort in soliciting private donations and applying for grants. There were successes and failures. The lack of money made it difficult to employ staff, and staff were necessary to manage clinic operations and oversee the volunteers. While the relationship between most of the clinics and the police was fine, several of the clinics—especially neighborhood clinics—were sometimes harassed by the police. The police department in Berkeley, California, raided the free clinic there and allegedly physically injured staff and patients. Clinics in Seattle, Detroit, Kansas City, Atlanta, and New Orleans reported instances of police harassment. Moreover, free clinics were essentially independent of one another. During the early years, there was no effective collective organization and only minimal communication among clinics (Schwartz 1971).

Of the 70 free clinics started between 1967 and 1969, 11 had closed by the end of 1970, and others were struggling to survive (Schwartz 1971). During the decade of the 1970s, as many as 300 additional free clinics were established around the country, but many of these, as well as many of the original clinics, did not endure. While no one was keeping close tally of clinic openings and closings through the 1970s, it is clear that more free clinics failed than survived. Nevertheless, most estimates of the number of free clinics in existence in 1980 are around 100–150, so there was a net increase during the decade (Weiss 1980). The establishment of more stable and more secure free clinics began around the middle of the 1980s, and this factor helped lead to a tremendous expansion in the number of free clinics during the 1990s and early 2000s. By 2004, there were an estimated 800 free clinics in the country, though fewer than 10 of the original 70 clinics were still in operation.

FIVE EARLY FREE CLINICS

In order to describe developmental features of the early free clinics, the remainder of the chapter focuses on five clinics that were started between 1967 and 1974 and still exist. The Haight-Ashbury Free Clinics, the Los Angeles Free Clinic, and the Berkeley Free Clinic were among the first generation of West Coast free clinics, although each has developed over the years in different ways; the Free Clinic of Greater Cleveland was one of the early midwestern free clinics; and the Bradley Free Clinic in Roanoke, Virginia, which began in 1974, was one of the first smaller-community, southern free clinics.

The Haight-Ashbury Free Clinics (San Francisco, California)

The Founding of the Haight-Ashbury Free Clinic

The conditions that led to the creation of the Haight-Ashbury Free Clinics, popularly regarded as the first clinic that embodied the clinic traits described in chapter 1, had been percolating for many years. The Haight district of San Francisco, centered around the intersection of Haight and Ashbury, was a low-rent Victorian neighborhood heavily populated by students. By the mid-1960s, it had become an oasis for artists, poets, writers, musicians, and hippies—a counterculture haven.

On January 14, 1967, a "Human Be-In" was organized in Golden Gate Park, just north of the Haight-Ashbury district, to protest a new law in California that banned the use of LSD. LSD had first been used in the United States in 1949 as a treatment for severe psychiatric problems that were resistant to other therapies. It was also found to aid cancer patients in dealing with their physical pain and psychological distress. It became best known, however, for its hallucinogenic properties and was a favorite among many hippies. Two San Franciscans, Allen Cohen (who ran a hippie magazine, the *San Francisco Oracle*) and Michael Bowen (an artist), organized the Be-In as a means to bring together radical social activists (especially from nearby Berkeley) and the "Hashbury," mostly nonpolitical hippies (Powis 2003).

> The Human Be-In stunned national media. Compared to such mammoth gatherings as Woodstock [in 1969], it was a piker. But it was the first time that thousands of psychedelic people, acid heads or simply "heads" as they were then called, gathered in one place at one time, and they were all just as amazed as the reporters. A new age had dawned! About 30,000 people in beads, flowers, peace paint, and some of them in nothing at all, were blowing the lid off America with Joy, Love, and Psychedelic Sound. Their philosophy boiled down to one word that appeared even on the nation's stamps: LOVE! As the news spread around the country with the speed of millions of television tubes, a trickle of young people with smiles, flowers, and backpacks became a stream, and then a torrent, complete with reporters, television crews, and sociologists. . . . By March, 1967, various groups within the community were reporting that Haight-Ashbury had filled beyond anyone's expectations. They predicted that at least a hundred thousand young people would flock to the district when school was out. (Seymour and Smith 1986, 18)

The city government reacted strongly and harshly. The mayor of San Francisco, John Shelley, warned outsiders that they were not welcome; the local bus company was requested to reroute its buses around the Haight district, and young people were prohibited from entering the park with a sleeping bag. Extra police were assigned to the area.

Within the Haight district, community activists began gearing up with services that would be needed by the influx of young people. An information and referral service was set up in one flat; an emergency housing program was set up in a church basement; a home and counseling center for runaways was created in an old house. What clearly was needed, but what was not available, was a health center targeted to the needs of the young people. The city proclaimed that they would need to use existing private facilities, but both a lack of funds and discouragement with the manner in which drug problems were treated in these facilities meant that an alternative was necessary.

Two individuals were especially important in creating that alternative. Robert Conrich, thirty-one years old at the time, son of a San Francisco

architect, a former private investigator, had dropped out of society's mainstream after taking LSD. He envisioned starting a private medical facility that
would treat adverse reactions to hallucinogenic drugs and provide care in a
nonjudgmental atmosphere. He hoped to become the administrator of the
clinic, and he approached a friend, a twenty-seven-year-old toxicologist
named David Smith, to become the medical director (Seymour and Smith
1986; Sturges 1993).

This fortuitous connection initiated events that ultimately led to David
Smith becoming the first visible leader of the free clinic movement. At the
time of the contact, Smith was chief of the Alcohol and Drug Abuse Screening Unit at San Francisco General Hospital, a unit that specialized in humane
and nonpunitive counseling and psychotherapy for drug users. In addition,
he was in the process of completing a postdoctoral fellowship in pharmacology and toxicology at the University of California at Berkeley and was
participating there in a pharmacology research group (studying hallucino-
gens and amphetamines) under the supervision of Dr. Frederick Myers. His
interest in Conrich's proposal also was triggered by conversations that he
had had with Florence Martin, an African American nurse, who had told him
about her experiences with a medical clinic that had been opened in the
Watts section of Los Angeles after the 1965 riot there. Part of the appeal was
the fact that the clinic had become a neighborhood center that was able to
marshal some political influence for improved health programs (Sturges
1993).

After planning for months, Smith and Conrich rented an empty dentist's office in the heart of the Haight district and set up an on-site conference to assess the interest of volunteers in supporting the clinic. When a large number
of both health professionals and street people showed up to express their
support, Smith and Conrich decided to go for it. Furniture was donated as
were other supplies including paper towels and toilet paper. Area hospitals
gave no-longer-used equipment, including an 1890 pneumothorax machine.
Pharmaceutical houses provided drug samples. On opening day, no one was
sure what to expect, but 50 people were in line when the clinic opened, and
more than 250 people were seen in the first day (including more than forty
cases of sexually transmitted diseases and fifteen cases of hepatitis) (Sturges
1993; Seymour and Smith 1986). David Smith recalls:

> If you saw this street with several thousand people, there was music all over the
> place, all sorts of kids in the waiting room having bad trips. I have lived in this
> neighborhood for forty-one years and really what we did was a crisis response
> to bad trips. There was relatively little long-term planning. We did have a phi-
> losophy that health care is a right and not a privilege, that love means care. That
> brought us together. Two things distinguished the line leading into the clinic
> that afternoon and evening—its diversity and its length. Most of the prospective
> patients strung around the corner of Haight and Clayton were young flower

children and beats and older hippies wearing beads and buckskins who had not seen physicians in months. Some came with their commune-mates, made music together, and passed out flowers. Others stood quietly, cradling infants to their breasts. Several dozen patients were spilling into the hallway, lining up outside the single toilet or drinking water from the bathroom sink. It was a madhouse. And it was an exciting day! (Sturges 1993)

Two days after the opening, the *San Francisco Chronicle* ran a very supportive article about the clinic. In it, David Smith discussed his hopes not only for helping the patients through bad trips but also for a meaningful aftercare program that would follow up on and monitor every patient. That, he said, required volunteer psychiatrists and psychologists. Money and volunteers came forward. Actors Hume Cronyn and Jessica Tandy offered to become volunteers and also contributed to the clinic. So did television actress Bonnie Franklin. Bill Graham, who was staging rock shows at the Fillmore Auditorium, visited the clinic, and, in what was a crucial step for the clinic, offered to stage benefit rock shows to raise money. Big Brother and the Holding Company (with Janis Joplin), the Charlatans, Blue Cheer, Creedence Clearwater Revival, George Harrison, Ravi Shankar, Led Zeppelin, and the Grateful Dead were among the groups who participated in these "Rock Medicine" benefits. (Seymour and Smith 1986)

The initial several months of the clinic were anything but easy. While the original intention of the clinic was to focus on all communicable diseases, it became obvious that most of the medical problems in the Haight were drug related. Eventually, the clinic would deal with a broad range of abused drugs—amphetamines, heroin, barbiturates, and prescriptive drugs—but the common drug problems in the first year related to bad trips on LSD. And, the medical establishment was, by and large, not trained to deal with these problems.

> The medical establishment at the time was woefully ill informed and badly equipped for dealing with psychedelic bad trips. Most health professionals did not understand the mechanisms involved. Seeing all psychedelic experience as instances of chemically induced schizophrenia, they often attempted to treat them with anti-psychotic drugs and physical restraints. They persisted in taking measures that exacerbated the situation instead of helping. As a consequence, it was common street knowledge that, aside from calling the police, the worst thing you could do for someone on a bad trip was take him to a doctor or an emergency room. (Seymour and Smith 1986)

The physical space of the clinic turned out to be too small. More than fifty physicians volunteered the first summer, but even that was not sufficient to handle the need. The city government was less than helpful. There were never enough funds. Conflicting philosophies existed about what it meant to be a "free clinic." In part, what held things together was David Smith's vision of the clinic.

The "Free" in Free Clinic refers more to a state of mind than to the absence of a cashier. Free means an entire philosophy of service in which the person is treated rather than his or her disease; it is an important distinction. In a free clinic the focus is on health **caring** for the whole person, on providing a service which is free of red tape, free of value judgments, free of eligibility requirements, free of emotional hassles, free of frozen medical protocol, free of moralizing, and last and least, free of charge. (Seymour and Smith 1986)

The Development of the Clinic

Despite the obvious need for the clinic and the existence of many supporters, the clinic (actually, by this time, renamed "clinics" to identify the multiple on-site programs) developed in fits and spurts. On several occasions, the clinics had to close down completely due to a lack of funds. At one point, a failed benefit concert left the clinics more than $20,000 in debt. A key administrator resigned after a heart attack. Changing patterns of drug use forced programmatic changes to a greater focus on heroin and barbiturates.

Over time, the clinics won grants from the National Institutes of Health and other government agencies. At times, these grants covered as much of the expenses of the clinics as possible and necessitated a division of organizational responsibilities into a variety of sections. Even during the lean times, the clinics pursued development of programs that responded to critical needs in the community. A dental clinic was added as was a women's needs center. In 1973, Rick Seymour was selected as "central administrator" for the clinics. Rick had been an English literature professor at Sonoma State University and had spent several years living in a rural commune in Mendocino. He had begun working at the clinics as a half-time secretary and janitor and had worked his way up through several positions. Rick shared in the vision of the clinics and used his writing skills to begin securing sizable grants. Within just a few years, the clinics had attracted four major federal grants (related to the War on Drugs), had an annual income of over $3 million, employed nearly a hundred people, had several hundred volunteers, and was providing 100,000 patient visits a year (Seymour and Smith 1986).

Then, in 1976, the federal government discontinued several of the grant programs that were funding clinic activities, and efforts were once again needed to reorganize the clinics. After considerable self-reflection and work with local and state politicians, the clinics developed strong working relationships with San Francisco City and County and with the state of California. These collegial relationships were beneficial in securing addition financial and community support.

The Free Clinics Today

Today, the Haight-Ashbury Free Clinics offer a wide array of services. The medical clinic provides primary medical care, comprehensive HIV care, chiropractic services, HIV and Hepatitis C testing, massage therapy, acupuncture, podiatry, physical therapy, and women's health services for more than 15,000 patient visits annually. In addition, clinic staff and volunteers provide medical care at rock shows and other concerts throughout the Bay area; provide mental health services to inmates of the San Francisco City and County Jail systems; offer substance abuse services through residential and outpatient drug treatment programs; sponsor a variety of research, education, and training programs; and provide a care program for the homeless.

The Los Angeles Free Clinic (Los Angeles, California)

The Founding of the Clinic

The Los Angeles Free Clinic was created in 1967—the Summer of Love—as the Albert Schweitzer Free Clinic to provide nonjudgmental medical care and draft counseling for the thousands of young people living in area parks and on the streets. Though several community activists and volunteers joined in the creation of the clinic, the lead was taken by two local psychologists who perceived the need for free medical services for the young people in the area. They rented a decaying storefront building, attracted many volunteers, began seeing patients . . . and were promptly reported by the *Los Angeles Times* to be lacking in professional credentials. By January 1, 1968, the board of directors quickly reorganized the clinic as a nonprofit corporation called the Los Angeles Free Clinic. The clinic was reestablished with a democratic structure with a coordinating council of representatives from multiple areas of service. Frances Helfman, who has volunteered at the clinic since these early days and served in a number of positions, recalled:

It was a time of social unrest, much psychedelic drug experimentation, and many college students coming to Los Angeles and San Francisco. Young people began pouring into the clinic with upper respiratory infections, sexually transmitted diseases, and unwanted pregnancies, and the free clinic was there for them. The doctors were young, and many were residents. Nobody was saying, "You rotten kids." They were accepted for whatever they were doing, and that was it, and they could get medical care, and they could get counseling services. We were considered outsiders doing something off the beaten track, and many did not want anything to do with the "hippie clinic"—a name that stuck for several years. We became experts in adolescents. Then, there was a gradual change to many, very intelligent, highly educated young people who were coming through. They were experimenting with drugs, they did not want to go into the army, and they were afraid of white supremacists. As the years went by, we noticed that the clients were getting younger and younger and younger, and then we started to get the high schoolers, we started to get youth who had run away from home. Working in those days was very stimulating, very exciting, and very sad. A lot of kids—"throwaways" they were called by society—had been thrown out of their own homes.

But it was a constant struggle to have enough money to keep the clinic open and to provide for the medical needs of the young patients. Clinic staff and volunteers frequently solicited gifts from wealthy philanthropists, often those with connections to the entertainment industry, and sometimes received surprise gifts, as occurred one day when Elvis Presley walked in with a $10,000 donation. However, the clinic survived mostly because of the efforts of the volunteers.

The Development of the Clinic

By the early 1970s, the hippies had begun to disappear, but the diversity of people in Los Angeles with critical needs for medical care continued to be reflected among clinic patients. The clinic continued to provide care for the homeless, for runaway youths, for immigrants, and increasingly, for the working poor. The clinic wanted desperately to avoid accepting government funds—an issue that the board debated on many occasions—and wanted to avoid instituting any fees for services, but more money was needed to run the clinic.

Though funds were continually scarce, the mood of the volunteers remained upbeat. As has occurred in free clinics around the country, the perception that good work was being done and that people's lives were genuinely being touched sustained optimism even when funds were short. There was evident pride that the free clinic was a site in which physicians could provide compassionate, holistic care and not have their attention focused on completing insurance forms and on regulatory controls. It was a type of throwback to the way medicine was once practiced and the way in which many of the volunteer physicians wished to be able to practice.

There was also recognition that more funds could expand the number of services provided. In 1973, Mimi West, a board member who held a master's degree in social work and whose husband had just been hired as a writer on a new CBS sitcom, *All in the Family*, founded a fund-raising arm of the clinic—The Friends of the Los Angeles Free Clinic.

I was so taken with what was happening there, how poor they were. There was never any money for rent. The Smothers Brothers paid the rent for a number of months. And, Lenny Somberg, the clinic director [who was tragically killed in a burglary at the clinic] only got $100 a week, if he got paid at all. . . . I began to nose around to find out why there was no money and no plan. And when I approached leaders in the community, I found out that most of them knew about the clinic and knew it did good work, but no one had asked them to help. (*Los Angeles Times* 1997)

Through the funds generated by the "Friends," clinic services expanded. Included among the new services was a High Risk Youth Program for homeless and runaway teens, a program that was created in a joint effort with Children's Hospital. In the mid-1980s, when the main clinic building could no longer house the necessary facilities, West spearheaded a capital campaign that raised $2.3 million dollars in just eighteen months. Support was generated throughout the community, a sign of the increased legitimacy of the clinic, and supporters in the entertainment industry were especially helpful in sponsoring fund-raising events. A new (the current) building was opened in 1990, and a second building (for the High Risk Youth Program) was added in 1992. The three-story main building enabled the clinic to offer more comprehensive services than ever.

The Free Clinic Today

With more than 2 million uninsured residents in Los Angeles County and with the magnetic force of Hollywood in attracting teenagers on the run, health care needs have continued to mount. Through the 1990s, the clinic board continued to revisit the idea of accepting government program funding, and by the late 1990s, the difficult decision was made to cross that threshold. Joseph Dunn, executive director of the clinic, points out what a profound change it was and continues to be:

The challenge is managing the cultural change that needs to take place in an organization like this for business functions to be integrated in a way that provides the financial stability but does not allow the core mission to vanish. That's kind of it in a nutshell. It is putting into place a discipline and infrastructure that have not been a part of the clinic. It is like going from a make-do organization in which everybody gets together and has a party or dinner and raises the money, and then next year, doing it all over again versus an organization that is no less under the gun from funding agencies than a hospital. We have to provide the same level of care and quality that everybody else does. We get the audits; we get the surveys; the Department of Health cares just as much about what we do as they care about someone else not serving our population. So we have to adjust in a way that allows us to be successful without abandoning our ability to serve those who come to our doors.

Today, the Los Angeles Free Clinic has an annual budget of $8 million, employs more than eighty full-time and part-time staff members, and has more than 600 volunteers. A comprehensive roster of services, including complete primary care, dental care, chronic disease management, family planning, HIV testing and counseling, diagnosis and treatment of sexually transmitted diseases, and women's health care (for example, breast cancer screening, pregnancy testing, and menopausal care) are provided for 70,000 patient visits per year.

The Berkeley Free Clinic (Berkeley, California)

The Founding of the Clinic

Although the founding of the Berkeley Free Clinic was in response to many of the same social forces that led to the creation of other clinics during these years, from the beginning the clinic has followed its own and somewhat different course. A paper written by Elena (1998), a clinic volunteer, describes the roots of the Berkeley Free Clinic:

> Prior to the social movements of the 1960s and 1970s, options for health care were basically limited to "fee for service" arrangements with private physicians and hospitals. Entire groups of people were either economically or culturally excluded, and the authority traditionally granted doctors reinforced many people's sense of alienation from their own bodies, and dependence on a system that did not serve them. With the heightened awareness of poverty and social injustice that arose from the New Left, civil rights and anti-war movements, activists began to see health care as one of several arenas for organizing for broader social change. They began developing "alternative institutions" as ways both to provide for society's basic needs, like health care, food, and housing, as well as to model a more egalitarian form of social organization. Hundreds of food co-ops, cooperative houses, and community health care clinics were organized during this era. The Berkeley Free Clinic is rooted deep within this context of struggle.

On the heels of the establishment of the Haight-Ashbury Free Clinic in San Francisco in 1967, several community residents in Berkeley began to strategize about creating a clinic there. Berkeley was very much in the national eye at this time as attention was often riveted on the University of California at Berkeley, the birth of the Free Speech Movement there, and the intense local activities of the Black Panthers and antiwar activists. In May 1969, the struggle over People's Park (and whether it could be used as a home base and sleeping quarters for young people and the homeless) erupted into a riot.

> Hundreds of people were injured, and an emergency field hospital was set up on the second floor of the McKinley School at Haste and Dana (now a UCSA housing complex) to treat riot victims. According to Scottosaurus [a long-time,

very dedicated clinic volunteer], police barged up the stairs hunting for escaped rioters, throwing a medic and an x-ray machine down the stairs. And so the clinic was born. (This also helps explain some practices which might otherwise seem idiosyncratic, like the use of pseudonyms or only using our first names.) (Elena 1998)

Many of the services at the new clinic were provided by Vietnam veterans who had been trained during the war as medics and who had now returned to the area. They provided around-the-clock emergency and "simple-complaints" service and a drop-in clinic that saw many young people for diagnosis and treatment of sexually transmitted diseases. A local counseling collective, the Radical Approach to Psychiatry or RAP collective, offered group counseling services. Some area dentists began accepting free referrals in their offices. A local information and referral service folded into the free clinic in 1970.

John Bartolome, now a staff member at St. Anthony Free Medical Clinic in San Francisco but a volunteer at the Berkeley Free Clinic in earlier years, explains part of the appeal of the Haight-Ashbury Free Clinics and the Berkeley Free Clinic:

> People who worked at the Haight and at the Berkeley free clinics were very hip, they were people to whom young people could relate. They did not have barriers around clothing and hair. They had people there who looked like hippies—and they were the physicians. But they came in to work with the people, and the kids could relate to them and could hang out . . . it was a very informal atmosphere. That's why they were very grass roots in their approach. There was not the formality or the division of lines between themselves and the people they were serving.

The core values of the clinic were included in its articles of incorporation. Medical care was to be offered for free (the motto of the clinic continues to be "Health Care for People not Profit"). Services were to be provided mostly by lay volunteers (who develop skills in a required apprenticeship program) under the supervision of health care professionals. On one hand, this limits the kinds of services that can be provided to mostly primary care, including conditions such as colds, coughs, sexually transmitted infections, skin concerns, bladder infections, stomach problems, and tuberculosis tests. Through an in-house dispensary, prescription and over-the-counter medications are provided. But, on the other hand, this enables the clinic to offer holistic care in a strongly supportive, nonjudgmental spirit.

> We try to provide a peer environment in which people are comfortable sharing information. Even when we see clients for things like a bladder infection, we ask about areas such as sexual health, overall stress level, diet, general concerns, other health concerns, housing, a job, information for their kids, so we

really offer a holistic approach. On average, our appointments are about an hour or hour and a half long, so that involves a lot of education. Most people come away with a lot of information and feel a lot better. (Sairah Husain, Coordinator of the Information and Referral Collective, Berkeley Free Clinic, Berkeley, California)

Perhaps the other most notable feature of the clinic is its commitment to collective organization. The right to participate in formal decision making about the clinic is granted to everyone who has volunteered at the clinic for at least two months. In the early days, however, the voice of the military-trained medics, due to their medical training and key position among the creators of the clinic, was especially powerful. This began to change in late 1970 when a group of thirty women formed a women's health collective. They requested use of the facility on one day each week to offer a clinic focused on women's health needs. The women's clinic quickly became very popular among patients and, at its peak, attracted more than 120 volunteers (Elena 1998).

The women's health collective brought a strongly feminist theoretical framework to the clinic. Their goals were not just about providing free health care, but to demystify medicine, de-professionalize doctors, and promote preventative medicine. They wanted to help women reclaim our bodies emotionally from "experts" and learn technical skills to care for ourselves. This new focus had a profound effect on the clinic's development and continues as a central part of the clinic's philosophy. (Elena 1998)

Tension between the medics and the more antiprofessional, collectively oriented feminists escalated, and many of the original medics left the clinic. Although the Women's Health Collective quickly outgrew available space at the clinic (and left for their own site in 1973), their impact was significant and lasting on internal organization. Clinic services became divided into sections, such as group counseling and information and referral; each section has a coordinator; and each section has periodic meetings at which all volunteers have an equal vote. There are also four (or however many are needed) all-clinic meetings each year, with each volunteer having a vote. It is common, even in collective organizations, for some informal authority to emerge, and the very small number of paid staff members (all of whom have also been volunteers, and some of whom volunteer at the clinic beyond their paid hours) and those who have been with the clinic the longest are in position to have more institutional knowledge and represent a type of leadership. But the collective organization approach is firmly in place, and the clinic does not have any full-time staff members. When I first contacted the clinic about visiting and interviewing key individuals, I spoke with David Kroman, a dedicated volunteer with more than nine-years' experience. He was very helpful to me and took my request to a meeting of the volunteers to determine if the clinic would participate in the project.

The Development of the Clinic

As the clinic moved through the 1970s and 1980s, staff and volunteers continually addressed clinic organization, clinic leadership, and the appropriateness of utilizing a larger number of paid personnel. In 1973, the paid workers began calling themselves an "administrative collective" and took on an increased presence in the clinic. They negotiated some government contracts, and these contracts typically had accountability requirements that necessitated the hiring of more staff. Changes in state law in the regulation of medical personnel in the mid-1970s required strengthening of the training program and new clinic protocols. However, in the late 1970s, tax limitation initiatives in California significantly decreased funds for the clinic. In a time known as "the Big Split" in the clinic, the budget was halved, the administrative collective was abolished, and most of the paid workers resigned. These funding pressures continued through the 1980s. The crisis intervention service was scaled back, the dental section was closed, and the defunct RAP Center struggled to re-create itself with more of a focus on individual counseling.

Nevertheless, something kept the spirit alive during these difficult transitions. David Kroman refers to it as a "sense of duty to the patients." It is the perception that, although the clinic may not be making a huge dent in the problem of inaccessible health care in the country, it is making a huge difference in the lives of some people. As David Kroman says:

> You do not have to save the world in order to make a difference in someone's life. While modern-day Western society encourages self-focus and not altruism, the clinic continues as a center for giving to others.

The Clinic Today

The clinic has achieved greater stability in the last decade. Currently, the clinic is organized around seven different sections: information and resources, general medical services (including a women's gynecological clinic), a dental clinic, HIV prevention services, a gay men's health service, hepatitis services, and peer counseling. Each is headed by a nominally paid coordinator and staffed by volunteers (the clinic has more than 200 volunteers). Volunteers are required to complete a rigorous three-month training process (eight hours per week) with a minimum one-year volunteer commitment that follows. The population served includes low-income residents, students, people between jobs, and the homeless. They come because no fees are charged, no qualifying screening procedure is used, confidentiality (anonymity for HIV testing) is assured, and patients are encouraged to become partners in their own care.

> Our services are very client-oriented, we put the client first, their needs first, we try to make sure that all of their needs are met, and it's a really gratifying experience as a provider working at a peer level. People come out of appointments with a much better feeling about themselves, and they come out happier knowing that someone cares. They have a better sense of what is going on in themselves, and they feel less scared, less frustrated. (Sairah Husain, Coordinator of the Information and Referral Collective, Berkeley Free Clinic, Berkeley, California)

The Free Clinic of Greater Cleveland (Cleveland, Ohio)

The Founding of the Clinic

As were the other hippie drug clinics, the Free Clinic of Greater Cleveland was born out of the 1960s counterculture and the greater use and abuse of drugs during that time. Many individuals, especially teenagers and young adults, in the Cleveland area had a great need for medical services but felt distanced from existing help systems. Their alienation from medical services and the consequent lack of attention to their medical problems was recognized by a group of community activists and young medical professionals in Cleveland, and they got together to talk about solutions. Several of the individuals involved in these conversations had been with the Haight-Ashbury Free Clinic during its start-up in San Francisco and were able to share their personal experiences. When members of the Cleveland foundation community began sitting in on the meetings, a full-blown planning process was under way.

The clinic originated as an "almost 24–7" crisis hotline staffed by volunteers who had undergone a crisis intervention training program. The hotline was successful, but it also brought to light the need for a comprehensive medical clinic. In June 1970, the free clinic was created in a three-story house that was located across from University Hospital's emergency room. That was somewhat ironic because many of the young individuals in the area had indicated that they did not feel comfortable with the way that they were treated in the emergency room. There, the protocol was to notify the police in case of a drug overdose, and that deterred many from seeking care there. In a larger sense, health services throughout the community were simply not prepared for the new rush of problems engendered by drug abuse.

> The health care system was based on a different ideology. The counterculture was a square peg in a round hole. In the medical community, few people had the breadth of knowledge of how to respond to drug overdoses or were able to

keep up with what was on the street or were able even to tell quickly the difference between an opiate overdose or a bad trip on LSD which requires very different tracks. Some had that knowledge, and they were part of the free clinic effort. (Marty Hiller, Executive Director, Free Clinic of Greater Cleveland, Cleveland, Ohio)

The clinic started as a walk-in medical and counseling clinic and as a liaison with other services in the community. When it became clear that the clinic was well matched to the need, other resources in the community aided the clinic. Several of the major hospital systems came on board—allowing people the opportunity to volunteer at the clinic and to be insured while doing so, allowing the free clinic to go into the institutions to recruit, providing drug samples, and referring patients. The private funding community became an important source of dollars; the Cleveland Foundation, the Gund Foundation, and several family foundations were important contributors. Various religious organizations melded their efforts into the work of the clinic.

However, key doubts about the clinic remained in the law enforcement community. They had to be convinced that the clinic was actually treating patients and not being used as a conduit for drug sales. The clinic's board of directors, especially a prominent attorney who was board president for seventeen years and several key individuals from area hospital systems, were important in convincing those in law enforcement about the legitimacy of the clinic.

The Development of the Clinic

In 1975, the clinic moved to a much more spacious building that was close to East Cleveland and the near Heights area, a location that increased easy access for a more diverse population. Through the 1970s, clinic services expanded in a variety of ways, financial support for the clinic increased, the building was purchased, and the most glaring needs in the community began to change. This was a point that almost all of the early clinics faced, but they dealt with it in different ways. The Free Clinic of Greater Cleveland was among those that allowed its primary service population to evolve. What had started as a counterculture organization, and had attracted many volunteers who identified with the counterculture, increasingly became the safety net for the working poor and the medically uninsured and underinsured. Care was taken not to exclude the original target population, although it was clear that more community programs had been created to provide those services; but the focus swung toward those who lacked access to private medical care.

This was a difficult period of time for many of the early free clinics, and it was the point in time when many of the early clinics closed their doors.

Others, like the free clinic in Cleveland, went through an uncomfortable transition, but one that enabled it to position itself to continue to focus on community needs. By the mid-1980s, the clinic had regained a solid financial footing and had begun once again to expand services. One of the first anonymous HIV testing programs was created in 1986; a non-hospital-based outpatient treatment program combining medical and mental health services was established in 1988; and the first syringe exchange program in Ohio was started in 1996.

The Clinic Today

With an annual budget of approximately $3 million, the Free Clinic of Greater Cleveland now provides services for over 20,000 patients each year. In 2002, the clinic moved into a new, modern facility adjacent to the former building. More than 600 volunteers, including physicians, dentists, psychiatrists, psychotherapists, midlevel practitioners, nurses, laboratory technicians, social workers, and lay volunteers provide a wide range of medical and mental health services. Services provided include evening walk-in clinics; adult primary care including treatment for hypertension, diabetes, asthma, high cholesterol, and gynecology; women's annual exams and Pap smears; men's and women's sexually transmitted infections; birth control; physical examinations; HIV; dental; substance abuse; mental health; and a variety of other specialty services.

While the working poor have become the primary group served by the clinic—almost three-fourths of the patients are employed—the clinic continues to see a diverse population. When asked about free clinic patients, Marty Hiller, the executive director, responded:

> It is for the guy who walks in the door in the middle of December, who comes into the walk-in clinic because he has a pain in his foot, and when they take off his shoes his toes are black. It's for the guy who comes in because he has been having headaches, and he needs to see the doctor to get something to help with the headaches, and he has a blood pressure of 180 over 130 or 240 over 130 which we had last week. In those sorts of circumstances the patient does not walk out of here, the ambulance comes to take him away. It is for the teenager who walks through the door because she is thinking about being sexually active, and she is not really sure what she wants to do about that, not even sure that she wants to. What they can do here is have someone to talk to. It is for the people who come here whose lives are, from one end to the other, precarious, and if there is a health problem that gets added to that equation, the whole house of cards can collapse. The people we see here are people who are trying to live their lives like anybody else, take care of themselves, take care of their families, make things a little better for the kids. It is just that for large segments of our population, as evidenced by the 20,000 or so people we see here every year, the cost of health care makes those kinds of aspirations impossible dreams.

The Bradley Free Clinic (Roanoke, Virginia)

The Founding of the Clinic

During the Vietnam War, Henry Bell, a young carpenter in Roanoke, Virginia, was assigned to fulfill his conscientious objector status at the Fan Free Clinic in Richmond. After fulfilling his responsibility, he returned home eager to help start a similar facility in the Roanoke Valley. He enlisted the help and support of his surgeon-father, Houston Bell, and the minister of his church, Dr. George Bowers of St. Mark's Lutheran Church. In turn, they attracted interest from others in the community, including a young medical resident from New York City, Dr. Richard Surrusco. A core group formed a board of directors, which met for a year to hammer out the structure of the clinic and clinic policies. Estelle Nichols Avner, who had been running a nursery school program, agreed to be a volunteer director.

St. Mark's Church donated rent free the bottom floor of an old 2,400-square-foot brick house in a relatively convenient area of town. The house had enormous charm (for example, high ceilings, brick fireplaces, and beautiful mirrors) but, of course, was not configured at all to be a medical facility. But the volunteers adapted, and the clinic opened in October 1974. The facility was staffed all day, but the medical clinic was open only on Tuesday and Thursday evenings. This was due in part to the desire to be accessible to those who worked during the day and in part to the fact that the clinic was volunteer-driven and used volunteers who came to the clinic in the evenings after they got off work.

The examination rooms were created by curtaining off sections of the living room. The patient waiting area was in the dining room, and when the chairs there filled up, on the front porch. The kitchen became a pharmacy; the pantry became a medical laboratory. Medical and social histories were done in small rooms, sometimes in converted closets. Most everyone thought it was wonderful.

> We had shower curtains on wires between the beds in the examining room. Going into a situation like that, you realize that you are going to have to be creative when you are going to do a Pap smear, and there is a shower curtain between you and the ten-year-old next door. We had the feeling of a little bit of a MASH unit. We did our best, but we knew that it was not going to be great. There was always a crowd in the waiting area and on the steps waiting to be seen. The need was obvious, that was the big thing. It was fun right from the start. (Kevin Kelleher, MD, Medical Director, Bradley Free Clinic, Roanoke, Virginia)

> In the early days, I used equipment at the free clinic that I am sure Doc Holiday must have used. I tell people that I learned more about emergency dentistry and pain relief dentistry there than I ever did in dental school. You are working in a situation where you don't have anyone to bail you out and you do what you have to do. (Vic Skaff, DDS, Bradley Free Clinic, Roanoke, Virginia)

The initial fear was that no one would come. Flyers were put all over town. On the first night, eight patients showed up. Twenty-five hundred more came the first year. After six months, Estelle became the paid director (and thirty years later is still the executive director), an event that perhaps everyone connected to the clinic still describes as the single most important reason for the success of the clinic. Protocols were developed on the run, as the clinic learned more about the needs of the patients.

> Nobody knew what the hell they were doing. There was no protocol, no sequencing, we just had to sit down and brainstorm. I remember one meeting at which we just sat down and asked who are the players, that if this is to be successful, who do we need to sign on—the medical community, the politicians, the general public? Most people are pretty decent, and they want well, and they want to help with those good things to the extent that their means—their time and their pocketbook—permit, so this was not an idea that wouldn't sell. (John "Lucky" Garvin, MD, former Medical Director and Board President, Bradley Free Clinic, Roanoke, Virginia)

The needs of the patients in Roanoke were not unlike the needs of those in the other early free clinics. Patients came in with every conceivable acute illness. Often, patients came in with conditions that were fully treatable but for which they had never been treated. While there are more programs today for children, in the early years, parents often brought their children for medical care for which they would not otherwise have had access. Many teens and young adults—trusting in the confidentiality of the clinic—came in for examination of symptoms of sexually transmitted infections. Many women came in to determine if they were pregnant. Periodically, patients with advanced chronic, degenerative diseases (like cancer) came to the clinic too late for cure. The biggest challenge, even then, was medications. Patients would come in, be seen by the physician, and be given a medication that might have cost twenty, thirty, forty or more dollars at that time— an amount that was not affordable. Calls for drug samples went out to local physicians, and the clinic volunteers often chipped in. But it was clear that the need was overwhelming.

From the beginning, securing support from physicians in the local medical community was key. There was confidence that volunteers from many sectors would come forward, but the doctors were the key. The initial reaction of the medical community in Roanoke—a relatively conservative community of about 225,000 people in southwestern Virginia—was very negative. Free medical care in Roanoke? A clinic for young, long-haired, drug-abusing, sexual disease–transmitting street people in Roanoke? Dr. Surrusco was called before the medical board of the hospital where he was serving as a resident and was grilled for more than an hour. These physicians had worked hard for their degrees and the idea of just giving medical care away for free was anathema. But, if there was going to be such a facility, they wanted to be certain that the professional medical community served as guardian. They asked questions about target population, clinic structure, ways of ensuring appropriate standards of care, and ways of ensuring that the patients seen had no other alternative for medical care.

They agreed to visit the facility. While the visit did not win overwhelming support, it did reduce most of the vocal opposition. Most visitors were convinced that people who really needed care were being seen. Two of the three local hospitals were still concerned about the loss of paying patients, but thanks in large part to Dr. John Garvin agreeing to be the medical director, his hospital, Lewis-Gale Hospital (now Lewis-Gale Medical Center), became a crucial early contributor to the clinic. Dr. Garvin invited some of the most well respected physicians at Lewis-Gale to tour the free clinic. They did so and then went back to the hospital and convinced the administrative hierarchy of its value. The hospital signed on to do laboratory work for the clinic for free. Years later, the other two hospitals also became important clinic supporters.

> With the medical community, we progressively signed on more voices with weight and propriety—people who were known for their propriety and devotion to medicine, and it became an exponential thing. It happened as more people with credibility signed on in principle and then signed on in practice. (John "Lucky" Garvin, MD, former medical director and board president, Bradley Free Clinic, Roanoke, Virginia)

Quickly after opening, the clinic realized there was a tremendous need for dental services. Patients were coming to the clinic and receiving treatment for their physical ailments (and even their mental health issues as volunteer professional counselors had come on board), but were often suffering from very serious tooth decay and, not uncommonly, excruciating pain. Two local dentists, Dr. David Black and Dr. Vic Skaff, had already been discussing the fact that many folks were unable to pay for their services. They discussed the possibility of seeing these nonpaying patients for free on one Saturday each month but decided instead to approach the clinic about creating a dental facility there.

Shortly thereafter, the free clinic created an on-site dental facility. It was sited in the old house's kitchen; it offered one dental chair that had been donated; the dentists brought their own instruments (and their assistants) from their offices; and they volunteered one night per week. The focus was on relief from pain, and many of the patients were in intense pain. Few had ever had ongoing dental care, they had little knowledge of dentistry, and they had multiple, serious dental problems. There was little that the dentists could do other than extractions. The local dental society had many of the same reservations as had the local medical society, so recruiting of other volunteer dentists went slowly.

The Development of the Clinic

Through the late 1970s and 1980s, the clinic constantly rearranged its facility to provide more usable space, add to its revenues in order to add to its services, to become better known, and to become more integrated into the community. More and more patients were seen. Important support from the local United Way was won as were some financial contributions from local governments, and increased giving, from small to very large donations, by local citizens and organizations. Other community organizations, such as the Council of Community Services, Planned Parenthood, the League of Older Americans, and a local crisis intervention center, helped out. And, more and more patients were seen. In 1989, a local philanthropist, Marion Via, gave the clinic $1 million (which was supplemented by an additional $900,000) to purchase a fairly new medical building whose occupants had moved to a larger space. (The clinic is now named the "Bradley" Free Clinic in honor of this philanthropist's father.) Nothing could match the charm of the old house, but the new building was a wonderful medical space that allowed more privacy, more services, more comfort, and more organization. It offered 9,000 square feet, nine examining rooms, four dental operatories, and a full pharmacy.

Services were expanded to include eight types of specialty care including ophthalmology, rheumatology, and psychiatry. Medical records were computerized, disease management profiles were created, and systematic vital statistics were maintained. In 1992, staff and volunteers formed the Free Clinic Foundation of America to provide support for communities wanting to start a free clinic and to facilitate communication among free clinics. A "How To" manual was published, and a national directory of free health clinics was compiled and distributed.

The Free Clinic Today

The Bradley Free Clinic has continued to grow, to become well respected within its community, and to help facilitate the development of free clinics in Virginia and in the United States. Estelle Avner has consulted personally with more than two dozen clinics in their formative stages, and several of the executive directors interviewed in this book give her much credit for helping them get started. Clinic staff and volunteers helped get a Good Samaritan law, which provides liability protection for volunteer health care workers, passed in Virginia. Dr. Kevin Kelleher, the clinic's medical director, has testified before the United States Senate on issues related to free health clinics and has published on free clinics. In 2002, the Bradley Free Clinic passed two milestones: it provided services for its 200,000th patient visit, and the total dollar value of services provided passed the $20 million mark.

3

The First Transformation in Free Health Clinics: An Increased Focus on the Uninsured and Working Poor

Tears were streaming down her face: "Somebody is going to help me just because I walked in the door, and they didn't even know I was coming."

(A free clinic patient)

THE EARLY YEARS

The initiative for starting the free clinic was the need for services by teens and young adults generally related to drug abuse and the sixties counterculture. Drugs were becoming more prominent then across society. Existing help systems did not know what to do with this emerging population, and often, what they did do alienated many of the people who needed help. . . . Many of these young people feared the protocol followed when overdose patients went to the emergency room. Frequently, police were called because it was a legal problem. There was an understanding that if you go to the emergency room, the police were going to be involved in your life, so these young people simply stopped going. (Marty Hiller, Executive Director, Free Clinic of Greater Cleveland)

As described in chapter 2, the origin of the hippie drug clinics—the majority of the early free clinics—was based on the perceived failure of mainstream medicine to provide adequate primary and specialty medical services for young, disaffected persons. Often, health care professionals and facilities failed to provide care in an emotionally supportive, nonjudgmental manner and failed to protect patient confidentiality. Individuals seeking care for drug-related problems, for problem pregnancies, for sexually transmitted infections, and for contraceptive services could not find available services and often felt mistreated when they did enter the medical system. The cultural chasm between the medical establishment and many of the young people in their teens and twenties was huge and resulted in many persons failing to obtain needed medical services.

It may be difficult from our perspective in the twenty-first century to look back at the late 1960s and early 1970s and fully appreciate what a serious medical crisis this was. Society was undergoing a major transformation, a large counterculture had developed, drug use was more prominent, and freer sexual relations often occurred without contraceptive protection. The array of drug treatment and rehabilitation programs and family planning programs that exist now had yet to be created or were in their infancy in most places. No matter how serious their medical problems, many young persons refused to see private physicians or to show up at hospital emergency rooms. Not infrequently, they experienced serious and sometimes contagious medical conditions such as hepatitis and sexually transmitted infections. The medical mainstream was not prepared for this tidal wave of change, did not respond well to it, and allowed a gigantic hole to be created in the medical care system. Many young people fell through the hole.

Neighborhood (minority) clinics also were created to respond to medical crisis—the inadequacy of accessible medical resources within minority communities. This was not a new problem in the United States, but it was an expanding problem in terms of the number of people affected, in terms of the recognition of the problem, and in terms of the determination by strong voices in the communities to do something about the problem. When free health clinics were established in minority communities, they were quickly overwhelmed by a backlog of unmet need. In these early years, both adults and children desperately needed access to primary care services for acute illnesses.

THE SHIFT IN FOCUS TO THE UNINSURED AND WORKING POOR

Free health clinics have undergone three major transformations from their early years until the present day. The first and perhaps most obvious of these transformations is the shift in target population to the uninsured—especially to the working poor. This is not to say that all free clinics have adopted this focus. Some free clinics in large cities continue to be a main medical provider for individuals experiencing drug-related health problems. Some clinics continue to target homeless persons and may be the only available community provider for them. Some clinics—especially in North Carolina—focus their services on providing needed medications. Some clinics see a preponderance of recently arrived immigrants to this country, including those who are undocumented. However, by far, the largest number of free clinics today have a mission of providing care for the working poor and for the uninsured. In many communities, these patients have been identified as being those in greatest need of medical care for acute illnesses and for chronic conditions such as hypertension, diabetes, heart disease, and asthma.

This important shift occurred as the late-sixties–early-seventies counterculture that helped shape many of the early free clinics diminished and largely faded away. American troops were brought home from Vietnam, and concern about being drafted was ended. The assassinations of Martin Luther King, Jr., and Robert Kennedy and the election and reelection of Richard Nixon as president and Ronald Reagan as governor of California and then president discouraged many of the young social activists. Some of the activist energy stayed alive, but as the counterculture generation aged their commitments often morphed into dedication to jobs within the system. While, for some, the articulated goals of the era were only a passing phenomenon, for others, they became the basis for new lives and new commitments. Clearly, however, the massive outpouring of young people into urban concentrations and the highly visible expressions of the counterculture declined.

This did not mean that all of the medical problems associated with countercultural life disappeared. The need for appropriate and respectful drug treatment programs has continued, as has the need for confidential educational and treatment programs regarding sexually transmitted infections, problem pregnancies, and contraceptives. However, a greater recognition of these issues has led to the development of an increased number of public and private programs targeted on these services. While the quality of new drug treatment programs and their ability to meet community needs vary, more money, more facilities, more qualified staff members, and greater effort have been put into drug treatment and rehabilitation. Additional family planning programs—like those run by Planned Parenthood—have been created and those already in existence often expanded from being education-only programs to offering clinical services. Typically, they offer low-cost, confidential, sensitively provided women's health care services including contraception, problem-pregnancy consultation, treatment for sexually transmitted infections, abortion (sometimes), and counseling. Individuals who once relied on free health clinics for these types of services have increased options, and often these options are in facilities that offer more clinic hours per week and an ability to focus on specific areas.

For some free clinics, these changes led to a perception that their primary mission was no longer needed—at least in such a dramatic way. Many clinic staff members and volunteers concluded that the clinic was no longer essential in helping to provide the needed services. Perhaps more commonly, some clinics simply lost some of their energy, some of their inspirational and driving leaders, and some of the community perception that they were filling a void in the health care system.

However, most clinics responded to these changing circumstances by refocusing their efforts. They viewed their mission as collectively acting to identify the largest holes in the health care safety net in their community and to marshal forces to address the unmet needs. As certain of the needs became addressed by other services, other needs became more pronounced, more visible, and more demanding of services outside the private care system. Free clinic communities around the country perceived that more and more individuals and families were going without needed medical care because they lacked health insurance and the financial resources to purchase private care. So, while the target population changed, the mission of targeting services to those in the community with the greatest unmet health care needs did not. As community-based facilities, free health clinics had the ability to shift their primary attention to the medically indigent. This overlapped to a large degree with the original vision of the neighborhood minority clinics—to provide free medical care services to those lacking financial access to the private care system.

BACKGROUND OF THE NEED

The United States Health Care System in Global Perspective

Countries around the world have created a diverse array of approaches for organizing their health care systems. The approach is usually influenced by a wide variety of factors including political factors (such as the general level of concentration of power in a central government), economic factors (such as the general type of economic system and the level and distribution of wealth), social factors (such as the reliance on formal organizations versus family for basic necessities), and demographic factors (such as the growth rate of the population). Cultural values also are important—especially the emphasis on personal versus social responsibility, attitudes about social inequality, and level of concern for the general public welfare and for those with the fewest resources. Sometimes, specific historical events (such as a very dynamic leader with strong views on health care or an economic recession that displaces large numbers of individuals) have an impact (Alford 1969; Lassey, Lassey, and Jinks 1997; Leichter 1979).

Despite the extensive differences among countries around the world, *all* modern countries—with the United States being the only exception—share the belief that people who are sick, regardless of their personal resources, should be able to get medical care—that is, medical care is a *right*. The United States is alone in taking the position that only people with sufficient resources—money or health insurance—have a right not to suffer needlessly from sickness. This position is often seen as being aligned with America's commitment to capitalism and private market forces (people will have more incentive to work hard and well if their health and life depend on it), with a culture that places higher value on individualism than community and higher value on self-interest than the general welfare, and with powerful groups in society that have successfully lobbied politicians to refuse to make a commitment to providing medical care for all persons.

The manner in which other countries guarantee access to health care varies considerably but generally follows one of three models. Some countries—Canada is a prominent example—provide *health insurance to all citizens*. Canada's system, which some in the United States routinely mislabel as being socialized medicine and routinely describe inaccurately, is basically a private medical care system. However, the national government requires all Canadian provinces and territories to establish a medical care system that provides universal health insurance coverage, access to comprehensive medical care services, portable benefits (individuals can be seen wherever they are in Canada), and public financing of the system. Funding for the system comes from both the national and provincial governments. To help control costs, Canada uses a process of "prospective budgeting"—that is, the budget for health care services is set at the beginning of the year, and providers must attempt to function within these limits. Given the amount of money that Canada budgets for health care, there are fewer high-technology pieces of equipment—for example, magnetic resonance imaging machines (MRI)—and fewer high-technology services available than in the United States. This is the reason that patients in Canada wait longer than patients in the U.S. for these services. But all persons can receive the services, and no one is barred from medical care due to inadequate financial resources.

Great Britain exemplifies a second approach, a *national health system*. Britain's "the National," as it is called, is based on government ownership of most hospitals and other health care facilities, employment of most health care providers, and extensive health planning. Patients can see specialists only upon referral by a general practitioner. Residents of Great Britain receive a card that entitles them to receive almost all medical care at no charge. As in Canada, patients do not receive services as quickly as is customary in the United States. Great Britain does have a small private health care sector, which means that those with sufficient financial resources to purchase private insurance can "jump the queue" and get services immediately.

The former Soviet Union and some Eastern European countries represent *socialized medical care*. In this type of system there is maximum centralization of authority in the national government and extensive structuring of the health care system. The Soviet Union's national Health Ministry was responsible for health planning, coordination of medical research, medical education, standards for medical practice, and formulation and allocation of the health care budget. The government owned all of the medical facilities and employed all of the medical providers. Patients had little choice of provider, and providers had little choice about accepting patients. As part of this government control, the health care system provided services to patients at no charge and encouraged patients to make frequent physician visits to monitor their health.

The United States Health Care System

The health care system in the United States is sometimes referred to as a *mixed-market* system because it is based on a private sector foundation but with significant public involvement. Today, business corporations (which now own many medical care services and facilities and insure patients); governments at the federal, state, and local levels; and, to a lesser degree, those in the health care field all play key roles in the system. It is an extraordinarily complex system that includes both for-profit and not-for-profit enterprises, both private (commercial) and government-sponsored (Medicare and Medicaid) health insurance, employer-provided and individually purchased insurance (in addition to government-provided), and a host of health-related organizations and agencies that are fully federally funded, partially federally funded, or receive no federal funding. Physicians may be self-employed or employed by a group or by a facility. They may be compensated for services directly by patients, by health insurance that is sold to the patient or to the patient's employer, by a managed care network, or by the government.

Advocates for this approach praise the fact that the U.S. has retained an essentially private care system often run to make a profit. They believe that competition leads to incentives to provide the best possible health care and for individuals to work hard to make money so that health care and other necessities can be purchased. Critics charge that a system motivated by profit is unlikely to always put the interest of patients first and that it ensures that many people not able to afford medical care often will go without needed services.

The United States system has many strengths, including the fact that it offers an extremely high level of technological care, and it includes a strong medical education system that produces highly qualified health care professionals. But the system often fails to get services to those in need. In 2000, the World Health Organization, using a sophisticated formula that includes many factors related to medical resources and health status, rated the U.S. system as being only the thirty-seventh best in the world. Another study evaluated the health care systems of twenty-nine industrialized countries on several important facets including provision of preventive care, health care use, mortality statistics, use of high-technology medicine, responsiveness of the health care system to disease trends, and stability of health care spending (Anderson and Hussey 2001). The U.S. fared poorly on most of the indicators and had failed to improve its worldwide ranking on a single one since comparable studies in 1960 and 1980. These ratings were given despite the fact that the U.S. spends much more money than any other country—in both absolute and relative terms—on health care. Life expectancy is higher in about twenty countries in the world than in the U.S., and infant mortality and maternal mortality are lower in about twenty countries. Medical bills are the most common source of bankruptcy in the U.S.—that does not occur in any other country. Many Americans are fearful of not being able to get services that are needed and do not think they could pay for medical care in case of a medical catastrophe. Surveys indicate that most Americans like and appreciate their physicians and other medical care providers, but they think the U.S. health care system has significant problems and is in need of major overhaul (Donelan et al. 1999). Surveys in other countries reflect a lack of respect for the fact that the wealthiest country in the world is the least generous with respect to ensuring that people can obtain medical care.

Public Insurance Programs: Medicare, Medicaid, and the State Children's Health Insurance Program

In the mid-1960s Congress enacted several pieces of legislation that were part of President Johnson's Great Society initiative and that represent an important government involvement in the health care system. Part of this initiative was a realization that millions of older Americans and millions of destitute Americans lacked the means to access the private medical care system. While these programs are much less comprehensive than programs developed in all other modern countries, their passage was an acknowledgment that the private medical care system was incapable of making health care available to all groups. In 1997, Congress created the State Children's Health Insurance Program (SCHIP) to provide select services for children in families with incomes too high to qualify for Medicaid but too low to be able to afford private care.

Medicare

Medicare is a federal health insurance program for people age sixty-five and older, for people with severe disabilities, and for people with end-stage renal disease. Part A of Medicare provides insurance for hospital care and is paid for by a mandatory tax paid by wage earners. Recipients are responsible for a deductible and copayments. Part B provides insurance for physicians' fees and is paid for by a premium paid by those eligible (including a deductible and copayments) and additional congressional appropriations. Part C of Medicare offers Parts A and B in managed care format.

Medicare is a generally well run program that now enrolls about 40 million individuals. Because contributions from today's workers help pay for

today's enrollees, the increasing number of people sixty-five and older relative to the number of people working combined with high health care costs
has kept the financial solvency of Medicare on somewhat shaky ground. To
address that, the premium for Part B and the deductibles and copayments for
both Parts A and B have continued to increase, so that out-of-pocket expenditures for Medicare enrollees have risen rapidly. Today, Medicare pays for
less than half of the total health expenses of those enrolled.

The biggest limitation of Medicare has been that it has not provided any
prescription drug benefit. Yet, the health and ability to survive for those with
chronic medical problems like heart disease, diabetes, hypertension, and
cancer—especially those with more than one of these medical conditions—
are dependent on taking the necessary drugs. Because medications are so
expensive, and because so many people in their later years need multiple
medications, many on Medicare have struggled to be able to afford drugs. It
is not uncommon for those sixty-five and older to forgo their medications altogether, to take only some of their medications, or to take the medications
less frequently than prescribed. One recent investigation found that some
seniors were so desperate for medications that they had asked for leftover
prescription drugs from family or friends who died, had sold precious pos-
sessions (such as a wedding ring) to pay for needed medications, and even
had taken medications (such as antibiotics) that had been prescribed for
family pets. Some have sought creative ways to be able to afford medications
such as purchasing them from Canada or another country, because prescription drugs are much more expensive in the United States than in other
countries (Barry 2003).

As an individual illustration of this serious problem: A sixty-six-year-old
woman in San Bernardino, California, a retired real estate broker, required
fourteen prescriptions to control her high blood pressure, thyroid problems,
and internal bleeding. She quit taking five of the medications, skipped doses
on some, and split pills on others to make them last longer. Her Medicare
HMO actually provides some drug coverage, so she is better off than most
Medicare enrollees. But the drug coverage is limited to $250 every ninety
days. Her most expensive drug costs $360 for a ninety-day supply. Even with
a required copay of $100, she is over her quarterly limit with just one pre-
scription with no coverage remaining for the other thirteen (Barry 2003).

In 2004 Congress passed a prescription drug benefit—Part D of
Medicare—to help with this situation. However, it is unclear to what extent
the bill—a compromised, watered-down version that seemed driven more
by securing votes in the 2004 election than a genuine commitment to the
elderly—will make a difference. At best, it will not come close to covering
the medication needs of those sixty-five and older, the amount of coverage
for each individual is based on a complicated formula that only Washington
politicians could devise, and it will use a system that will unnecessarily di-

vert valuable dollars to administrative overhead and to profit for the private insurance companies that will provide the coverage.

Medicaid

Medicaid is a federal-state program that provides health insurance for recipients of public assistance programs and for targeted groups of pregnant women, poor children, the disabled, and the aged. Today, Medicaid provides insurance to just over 30 million individuals. Although the value of helping the poor to access medical care is meritorious, Medicaid has been plagued by problems almost since its inception. It covers too few of the poor—only about 40 percent of those who are below the poverty level qualify for any Medicaid assistance. Of those who do qualify, there are fairly comprehensive services provided, especially for children, who account for half of all Medicaid beneficiaries. Payments to medical providers are relatively low, have been repeatedly scaled back, and now are at a level at which many physicians will not see Medicaid patients. Eligibility requirements, procedures, and services covered vary enormously from state to state, creating a very confusing system for those who move.

Despite all of these limitations, Medicaid is a very expensive program for both the federal government and state governments. It occupies about 12 percent of all state government spending and is one of the largest budget items for many state governments. In recent years, costs for the Medicaid program—like those for all health insurance programs—have been driven up especially by spending on prescription drugs. From 1990 to 2000, Medicaid drug spending increased from $4.4 billion to over $20 billion, an average annual increase of 16.3 percent. Disabled persons experienced an even greater annual increase in prescription drug costs during this time period—about 20 percent (Baugh et al. 2004). As state governments have increasingly faced budget shortfalls in recent years, there have been tremendous pressures to further tighten Medicaid spending. In fiscal year 2004, all fifty states and the District of Columbia implemented at least one action to control Medicaid spending (Kaiser Commission on Medicaid and the Uninsured). For example, Missouri cut coverage for more than 30,000 poor parents by reducing its Medicaid income limit from more than $15,000 to $11,750 for a family of three. Oregon cut coverage for more than 40,000 people. Texas took measures to reduce Medicaid enrollment by more than 100,000 people. Mississippi cut 65,000 Medicaid enrollees. In Alabama, a parent in a family of three with an income above $253 per month—the equivalent of working eleven hours per week at a minimum-wage job—makes too much to qualify for Medicaid assistance (Dedrick 2003).

For those who are extremely poor and receive Medicaid assistance, there has been clear improvement in health outcomes. But for those below the poverty level who do not qualify and those who are just above the poverty level, Medicaid has been of no help. Often, these are individuals who work full-time or at two part-time jobs at low wages. Their employers do not offer health benefits, and they make far too little money to be able to purchase a policy on their own. These individuals and families are often said to be too "rich" to obtain Medicaid and too poor to pay for private medical care and fall through the mesh of the so-called safety net.

The State Children's Health Insurance Program (SCHIP)

The SCHIP program, created in 1997, was an effort to create a federal-state partnership (similar to Medicaid) for children in low-income, uninsured families. States may implement their program by creating an entirely new program or by expanding the Medicaid program. Income eligibility varies from state to state, but is commonly set at 200 percent of the poverty level. States also have flexibility in determining what services are covered, but they must fall within federally established guidelines.

Enrollment in the SCHIP program grew quickly and steadily in the late 1990s and early 2000s to around 4–5 million in 2003 (membership numbers are counted in different ways by various agencies). Those enrolled have very favorably evaluated the program and services offered, but the same state budget woes that have negatively affected the Medicaid program have also harmed SCHIP. Several states have now taken actions to limit enrollment in their programs. As of January 2004, six states had frozen enrollment in their programs and had waiting lists of children waiting to enroll. Texas cut back its program. California is in the process of doing the same. Some states have added a premium to allow participation in the program.

KEY PROBLEMS IN THE UNITED STATES HEALTH CARE SYSTEM

The United States health care system has two overarching problems: very rapidly escalating health care costs and the fact that millions of people lack the financial wherewithal to pay for private medical care and do not have health insurance.

Huge and Rapidly Increasing Health Care Costs

In 1960, altogether, the United States spent about $27 billion on health care—about one dollar in twenty (5.1 percent) of the total amount of money spent on all goods and services (that is, the Gross Domestic Product or GDP). By 1980, the country spent more than $247 billion on health care—8.9 percent of the GDP. In 2003, health care expenditures reached $1,700 billion

($1.7 trillion)—more than 15 percent of the GDP and more than $5,800 for every American. According to recent projections, health care spending will double in the next ten years, reaching $3.4 trillion in 2013—about 18 percent of the nation's economy—that is, almost one dollar in every five. Year in and year out, increases in health care spending outstrip increases in all other sectors of the economy, and often health care increases double, triple, or quadruple overall cost-of-living increases. It is difficult to foresee ways that will restrain the expected increases, but many observers believe that, at some point, the health care system will implode (Cutler 2004).

There are many reasons for these startling increases, but three of the most important are new high-technology procedures, rapid increases in the cost of medications, and administrative complexity. First, newly developing and very expensive high-technology procedures are a major source of cost increases. Thus far, the country has accepted new technologies even though in some cases the benefits are marginal, the cost is huge, and few without excellent health care insurance can afford them. Second, each year, increases in the cost of drugs are the first or second most important component of increases in overall health costs. In the early years of the new century, prescription drug prices were increasing by more than 15 percent per year—an astounding rate of escalation. Drugs are much more expensive in the United States—where the government refuses to limit price increases—than in other countries where there are government controls. Third, the administrative complexity of the U.S. health care system is another responsible agent. It is estimated that more than 20 percent of all health care costs in the U.S. have nothing to do with clinical medicine—they are for administrative overhead. How does that compare with other countries? It is about twice as much. Yet, the U.S. has failed even to adopt something so simple as a uniform insurance form—something that could save billions of dollars annually in bookkeeping and billing expenses.

The Large Number of Uninsured Americans

While other countries make health care available to all citizens through government-enacted programs and policies, health insurance provision in the United States relies on (largely) voluntary-based, employer-provided programs. Most large businesses offer a health insurance policy to their employees as a benefit of employment. Typically, the employer pays for most of the cost of the policy for employees; in the United States, employers on average pay about 73 percent of the cost. Of course, policies cover only whatever services in whatever amounts that have been negotiated, and on certain expenses, patients must pay certain deductibles (an amount before the insurance kicks in) and pay specified copayments (an additional amount each time a service is used). While this system works for many, it is a complete failure for millions upon millions of Americans.

In the year 2000, 171 million Americans had health insurance through employer-provided insurance; 80 million people were covered by Medicare, Medicaid, and other public programs; 16 million people purchased their own health insurance, and more than 40 million people—about 17 percent of the entire population—lacked any form of health insurance. The public/private, employment-based system in the United States fails to make health insurance available to at least seven primary groups.

The system fails to provide coverage for individuals and their dependents who are unemployed.

The number of persons who are unemployed and the unemployment rate are, of course, in constant flux. In the year 2003, about 6 percent of America's labor force (between 8 and 9 million persons) were unemployed at any given time. These are individuals who do not have a job, are actively looking for work, and are currently available for work. Individuals who have become frustrated and stopped looking for work are not considered in the calculation of the unemployment rate. Because the primary way that health insurance is provided is through employment, those without a job are automatically cut off from this benefit.

These individuals can purchase a health insurance policy directly from a health insurance company, but this can be a very expensive option that can be fraught with difficulties. Coverage for existing medical problems may be excluded, and, if the problems are serious, an individual may not be able to purchase insurance at all (that is, those who need it most are least likely to get it). Twenty-nine states offer high-risk pools for those who are refused an individual policy. About 150,000 Americans receive coverage this way. But eligibility often is difficult, there may be waits for preexisting conditions, and there may be stringent caps on the amount of money paid out per year or over a lifetime. Only eleven states and the District of Columbia guarantee that all residents can buy health insurance no matter how sick they are.

The system, in some cases, fails to provide coverage for individuals and their dependents after retirement but before Medicare begins.

Some individuals are fortunate to have worked for an employer who continues to subsidize their health insurance even after retirement. But, due to the continued large increases in health care costs, many companies have discontinued this benefit, and most companies have significantly raised the percentage of the cost that must be borne by the retiree. In 2003, even among large companies, which tend to offer the most generous benefits, only about one-third still offered a retiree medical benefit, and the percentage is rapidly declining (two-thirds of companies offered retiree health benefits as recently as 1988). Of companies that do offer it, the percentage of cost that the retiree is responsible for has jumped in recent years from 0, 10, or 20 percent to 50 or 60 percent or more. For wealthy retirees, this may not be a problem. But for low-income retirees, who have just entered a time of significantly reduced income, significantly greater expense for health insurance is a heavy burden. If the annual cost of a health insurance premium is about $10,000 (which would be fairly typical for retirees in their early sixties), and the company subsidy decreased from 80 percent to 20 percent, the extra cost per month per retiree would be about $500, which would be very difficult for most retirees.

The system fails to provide coverage for individuals and their dependents during any transition period from one job to another.

Millions of Americans change jobs each year. Until recently, when an individual left a job, employer-provided health insurance ended. Coverage by health insurance provided by the new employer did not begin until the individual started the new job and often not for six months or twelve months after starting. This created a dangerous gap between coverage periods in which the individual and his or her dependents lacked health insurance.

In 1986 Congress passed the Consolidated Omnibus Budget Reconciliation Act (COBRA), that enables specified workers who have lost their jobs to continue their health insurance coverage for themselves and their dependents for up to eighteen, and sometimes thirty-six, months. To do this, however, the displaced worker is required to pay the portion of the insurance cost that she or he was paying plus the amount that was being paid by the employer. While this may be less than the cost of an individually purchased policy, it typically is very expensive—too expensive for many displaced workers to afford. Thus, an option was created that has been invaluable to some but not feasible for many others. In recent years only 20–25 percent of those eligible to purchase insurance through COBRA have done so, and almost all of those who have purchased it cite the high expense—routinely about $7,000 or $8,000 per year.

The system fails to provide coverage for part-time workers, including those who are working at two or more part-time jobs simultaneously.

Many workers are not able to secure a full-time position and work only part-time. In order to try and make ends meet, many take on a second part-time job and may work a total of more than forty hours per week. But employer-provided health insurance is a benefit given only to full-time workers. So, even though an individual may be working at a combination of part-time positions that total more hours than many full-time positions, no health insurance is provided. What's more, some employers (fast-food restaurants are a common example) intentionally hire workers at just under the number of hours per week that would make them full-time and eligible for a health insurance benefit. Stories of workers locked into this situation are not uncommon.

The system fails to cover the overwhelming majority of employees in small businesses, which are far less likely than large businesses to offer health insurance benefits.

Small businesses are treated very unfairly in the current system, and employees of small businesses suffer the consequences. Large employers have a distinct advantage in negotiating for health insurance coverage. Insurance providers recognize that especially costly procedures received by one or a few individuals in a large employee group can be spread across the entire group. Because the total cost of medical services received by many of the employees is likely to be less than the total amount of premiums paid in for them, part of the difference can be used to cover the higher costs incurred for others. Small businesses do not have this luxury. If one or a small number of employees in a small business have exceptionally high costs, there are not enough fellow employees to cover it. Therefore, health insurance companies routinely charge higher fees for policies for small businesses and raise their rates more sharply when high expenses occur.

The result of this pattern is that small businesses are much less likely to provide any health insurance coverage for their employees. In 2003, only 55 percent of businesses with 3–9 employees offered employee health benefits, while 98 percent of businesses with at least 200 employees offered health benefits (Kaiser Commission on Medicaid and the Uninsured). Moreover, the disparity is widening. From the perspective of the individual employee, is there any reason that an employee of a large company is more deserving of employer-provider health insurance than an employee of a small company? Of course not, but that occurs within the current system.

The system fails to provide coverage for individuals—and thus their dependents—who cannot afford the employee share of employer-provided health insurance.

The time when employers paid for the total cost of a health insurance policy for employees is almost gone (in 2003 only 4 percent of large employers, and virtually no small employers, still paid the full health insurance premium for employees). As mentioned earlier, the rapidly escalating cost of health care—and thus of health insurance—has reached staggering levels for many employers. Many have decided that they cannot afford to provide this extensive coverage, and so they have implemented mechanisms to have employees pay a greater share of the cost. This has been done in several ways. First, the services provided by the policy have been reduced, so that employees have to pay for some services that once were covered. Coverage for mental health service is often the first to go. Second, the amount of deductibles and copayments has increased because that reduces the cost of the policy. But employees are then responsible for paying a larger percentage of the cost of their care. Third, the percentage of the policy premiums paid by employees has been increasing and will almost assuredly continue to increase. Fourth, even in situations in which the company continues to pay a high percentage of the premiums for the employee, the amount contributed to cover the employee's family has begun to diminish.

According to surveys conducted by the Kaiser Foundation in 2003, only about two-thirds of employees today are covered by health insurance plans offered by their employer. Part of the gap is accounted for by individuals who are covered under a family plan offered by the spouse's employer. However, many individuals are opting out due to the cost of the employee share of the policy.

Employee groups have strongly resisted this cost restructuring. Over the last ten years, groups ranging from supermarket clerks to sanitation workers to public transit workers have gone on strike to protest the reduction in their health benefits. In some cases, compromise has been reached. But employers have made it clear that they are going to reduce the growth of their expenditures for employee health insurance, and that is a clear present and future trend.

Even persons with health insurance, when they get sick, are finding out that it often falls short. A recent study (*Consumer Reports* 2002) found that many insured persons now forgo needed medical treatment due to the cost. Of those with health insurance but earning less than $35,000 per year, more than 20 percent were unable to pay all of their medical bills, almost 20 percent failed to get a prescription filled in the previous year because of its cost, almost 20 percent failed to see a physician when sick, and about 10 percent did not see a specialist when needed and skipped a medical test or treatment. Even those with insurance and earning more than $35,000 per year sometimes forgo needed medical treatment because of the personal cost that would be incurred.

The system provides no coverage for individuals and their dependents who are in this country illegally.

Clearly, there are hundreds of thousands or more individuals in the U.S. who have crossed the border illegally. Many employers knowingly hire these individuals because they are willing to do jobs that others will not do, and because they are willing to work for less than the minimum wage. Often, they are paid under-the-table, so that their illegal status is not discovered. Of course, they are not provided with any health benefits. Working at a low wage and without health insurance means that it is very difficult for these people to afford medical care regardless of the seriousness of a disease or illness.

Other individuals are left out of the health care system.

The lack of financial resources—either money or health insurance—is the most common reason that individuals and families are left out of the private care system, but it is not the only reason. In some areas of the country—especially inner-city areas of large cities and rural areas—there are an insufficient number of medical providers. Some individuals—especially those newly arrived in the U.S.—have a very difficult time figuring out how to access the health care system. Some individuals—especially racial and ethnic minority group members and individuals whose illness may be caused by socially undesirable behaviors such as abuse of street drugs—still report negative experiences in the private care system and do not feel comfortable accessing care. Some individuals—especially young people—still lack confidence in the confidentiality of the private care system with regard to such matters as birth control, pregnancy testing, and sexually transmitted infections. Rarely can the homeless easily access private medical care. Each of these situations is important in and of itself. Nevertheless, in terms of numbers, the lack of financial ability to access the private care system is overwhelmingly the biggest source of the problem.

AMERICA'S UNINSURED POPULATION

Who are the Uninsured?

At any given time in the United States about one in every six people lacks any form of health insurance. In recent years this has been about 44 million people. However, over any two-year period, because many people go through periods where they transition from having to not having insurance, more than 80 million people are without coverage for at least some time. According to Families USA, 81.8 million people were without health insurance for at least part of 2002 and 2003. About two-thirds of these people were uncovered for at least six months, and half were uncovered for at least nine months. Lacking health insurance is something that can happen to anyone. While the number of uninsured fluctuates daily, the long-term trend is a steady increase, that is, there are more uninsured than ever.

While most people in the U.S. are aware that millions of people lack health insurance, many do not understand the gravity of the problem. A lack of insurance can and does occur for people from every walk of life. The following facts illustrate this pattern:

- Most people who lack insurance are employed. In recent years more than 60 percent of uninsured Americans have been in families with a worker who works full-time year-round, and additional 20 percent-plus are in families with a year-round part-time worker or a partial-year full-time worker. The perception that the uninsured are drawn largely from people who are unemployed is false.

- Being without health insurance occurs at all ages. People age twenty-five to thirty-four—in the early years of their careers, just beginning to get financially settled, often still shifting from job to job—are the age group most likely to be uninsured. The likelihood is then greatest for people age thirty-five to forty-four and forty-five to sixty-four.
- Most of the people who are uninsured are white. In recent years about two-thirds of the uninsured were white, about one-seventh were Hispanic, and about one-eighth were black. However, members of racial and ethnic groups are more likely than whites to be uncovered. During the 2002 and 2003 two-year period, almost 60 percent of nonelderly Hispanics were uninsured for at least some time. Why? Many Hispanics work in low-wage jobs for employers who do not offer health insurance benefits.
- People below the federally established poverty level (which was just under $19,000 for a family of four in 2004) are especially likely to lack health insurance. About one-third of these people lack health care coverage.
- The cost of purchasing health insurance is increasingly a problem for people in the middle class. The percentage of people earning incomes of $50,000 and more but who do not have insurance has risen over the last several years. Some commentators have suggested that this means that people are uninsuring themselves by choice rather than need, thus minimizing the problem. That misses the point in several respects. What this pattern reflects is that health insurance has become so expensive that even middle class families are struggling to pay for it. Many of the middle-class uninsured have children to support, home mortgages to pay, and college loans to reimburse, in addition to other basic expenses. Many are self-employed; many have been working only a few years and do not have large financial savings; many are taking care of elderly relatives. In such circumstances, suggesting that paying $8,000, $9,000, or $10,000 a year for a family health insurance policy is simply "choice" distorts the real situation. For those working for an employer that does provide health insurance, the increased cost borne by the employee in recent years has caused many to discontinue coverage. And, whatever the situation, going uncovered risks lifetime financial disaster in the case of catastrophic illness.
- While the lack of any health insurance is the key problem, being underinsured is also a very serious problem. While some policies offer high or reasonably high benefit levels, others have relatively low limits that can easily be exhausted in cases of prolonged serious illness. Some policies have high or very high deductibles, meaning that the individual or family must pay out-of-pocket the first $500 or $1,000 of medical expenses. For low-income families, this can be sufficient reason to defer medical care.

Who are the Working Poor?

The Definition of Poverty

There is not any one single completely adequate formula for determining the amount of money that it takes to be able to purchase life's necessities. Costs vary from region to region and locality to locality throughout the country; the cost of having two preschool children may be very different than having two kids in high school; and family living situations vary enormously. Since the 1960s, the United States has used a Department of Agriculture–determined formula to determine the poverty level. The formula is very straightforward but not at all precise. The amount of money that is necessary for a basic diet is determined and then that amount is simply tripled to calculate the poverty level. The underlying rationale is that low-income families should be spending approximately one-third of their income on food. A specific calculation is then made based on the number of persons in the family, and some variation is attached based on geographic location.

In 2004, the federal poverty level for the forty-eight contiguous states and the District of Columbia (it is higher in Alaska and Hawaii) was:

1 person in family—$9,310;
2 persons in family—$12,490;
3 persons in family—$15,670;
4 persons in family—$18,850.

Looking at this from a different perspective, a four-person family with one full-time worker making just over $10.75 an hour would be at the federal poverty level. If this worker made $11.00 an hour, the family would be above the poverty level and be considered "nonpoor."

The lowest-paying jobs in the United States are set at a wage level that is far below that in other industrialized countries. Beth Shulman, in *The Betrayal of Work: How Low Wage Jobs Fail 30 Million Americans* (2003), points out that the bottom 10 percent of American workers earn just 37 percent of the U.S. median wage, while comparable workers in other industrialized countries average between 60 percent and 76 percent of their country's median wage.

One of the serious limitations of the poverty level is that families on average now spend a considerably lower percentage of their disposable income on food. Today, expenses for housing, health care, job- and school-related expenses including child care, and transportation occupy a greater share of family expenses, and the typical family spends less than 20 percent of its budget on food. Thus, tripling the basic food diet cost produces only about 60 percent of family expenses. For those with higher incomes, this may not seem like an important difference; but for those whose incomes are in this range, it is a profoundly important inequity. Many social programs acknowledge this problem by allowing people who make 150 percent or 200 percent, or once in a while even more, to qualify for programs. That should be interpreted as basic fairness rather than largesse.

The term *working poor* refers to individuals who are working full-time or part-time, are on temporary layoff, or are unemployed and actively looking for work *and* whose families earn less than 200 percent of the federal poverty level. A common estimate is that we have 30 million people in "working poor" families in the United States.

Low-Wage, No-Insurance Jobs

The U.S. labor market may be broken down into three separate groups (Carnevale and Rose 2001). At the top are the "elite workers"—those who work in the professions, as managers, and in jobs that require technical expertise. These jobs typically require a college education, often a graduate degree, and are the most highly paid jobs by far. The "middle workers" are those who work in supervisory positions, as craftworkers, in public service positions such as police officers and firefighters, and many clerical workers. Though the educational qualifications for these positions vary, increasingly they require at least some college, an associate degree, or even an undergraduate degree. The third segment is the "less-skilled workers." These are jobs in factories, as farm and nonfarm laborers, as sales clerks, and as food and personal service workers. Most of these jobs require a high school education or something less than that. Some of these sectors, such as less-skilled manual laborers, are overwhelmingly occupied by males, while other sectors, such as less-skilled sales clerks and service workers, are overwhelmingly female.

The portrait of the low-wage workforce includes more diversity than might be expected. About 60 percent of low wage earners are in the third segment, but about 25 percent are in the middle segment, and about 15 percent are in the top segment. The latter two groups include many people who are self-employed, substitute school teachers, temporary clerical workers, and even some construction and landscaping workers (who often go through periods of underemployment and unemployment). Many less-skilled positions in the health care field fall into these two groups as might positions in the clergy, as artists, or as entertainers.

Some of the low-wage workers are secondary earners in the family and secure health insurance through their spouse. But that is not the most common pattern. Rather, these workers often are single parents or the only breadwinner in the family or at least a primary earner. If they have a spouse, the spouse frequently is also a low-wage worker and often neither of them receive health insurance from their job. The percentage of working adults (employed or self-employed) who do not have health insurance varies considerably from state to state. Minnesota, Hawaii, Maryland, and Iowa have the lowest rates of uninsured workers (all between 6 and 9 percent), while Texas (26.9 percent), Louisiana (23.2 percent), Mississippi (22.4 percent), and New Mexico (22.4 percent) have the highest rates (State Health Access Data Assistance Center).

Two recent events have created even more of a flow into low-wage jobs. First, in 1996 Congress enacted a significant change in America's public assistance programs with the Personal Responsibility and Work Opportunity Reconciliation Act. The thrust of the legislation was to move recipients of welfare into jobs rather than have them receive public benefits. This welfare reform occurred at a time when the economy was coming out of a downturn, and many new jobs were being created. Therefore, many individuals—primarily single-parent women—entered the labor force, the number of individuals receiving public assistance decreased (by more than half), and many declared the effort a success.

Unfortunately, too little consideration was given to the types of jobs into which these individuals were moving and to the overall consequences for their lives and families. Overwhelmingly, the jobs that they entered were less-skilled, low-wage positions that paid little more, if any more, than the amount of assistance they had been receiving, and few of the positions offered employer-subsidized health insurance. Many were able to find full-time employment, but others obtained only one or two part-time jobs. Though the wages were low, in some cases they moved the family above the threshold for qualifying for Medicaid, so the family entered the ranks of the uninsured. Other expenses—such as work-related expenses (it is estimated that about one-third of low-wage workers do not have a car) and child care expenses—were also added to the family budget, making it more difficult than ever to make ends meet. When the direction of the economy reversed in the early 2000s, many jobs were eliminated, and those who had just entered the workforce in the late 1990s were especially hard hit.

Forecast for the Number of Uninsured

The number of people in the United States without any health care coverage is likely to continue to grow. Almost all of the factors that influence that number point to continued increases. Health care costs are likely to continue to escalate, putting insurance out of reach for more and more people. Many forecasters predict that in the coming years health insurance premiums will increase at more than three times the rate of wage increases. Employers are almost assuredly going to continue raising the percentage of health insurance premiums paid for by employees and in many situations will be negotiating for policies with higher deductibles, higher copayments, and fewer services covered. Employees will be in the position of paying a higher percentage of a higher premium for less coverage. States across the nation are focused on reducing expenditures for Medicaid, meaning fewer people will be eligible and those who are enrolled will be covered for a smaller percentage of medical care costs.

THE CONSEQUENCES OF NOT HAVING HEALTH INSURANCE

The lack of personal financial resources to pay for private medical care and the lack of health insurance have a profound effect on the health of individuals and families. Studies have shown that people without health insurance are less likely to seek preventive medical care such as medical checkups (especially Pap smears and mammograms for women and prostate cancer screening for men) and immunizations. They are more likely to try to get through illnesses on their own without seeking a medical provider. If they do see a medical provider, they often have waited until they have become very sick, their health is more threatened, and in some cases such as patients with cancer or diabetes, the benefits of early detection are lost. They are less likely to have a regular source of medical care and more likely to see a different provider on each visit. They are less likely to receive mental health care. They are less likely to receive dental care. They are less likely to receive care from primary care physicians and are especially unlikely to receive care from specialists. They are less likely to be admitted to a hospital but are sicker when they are admitted. Despite this, they receive fewer expensive medical treatments while in the hospital and often are deprived of the benefits of medical technology (even when controlling for need, the uninsured are less likely to get clearly beneficial procedures such as heart bypass surgery, cataract surgery, and treatment for depression) (Schriver 1999; Friedman et al. 2002; Giled and Little 2003).

These negative health patterns occur among children as well as adults. Studies have determined that uninsured children are only one-sixth as likely as insured children to have a usual site where they receive health care. Uninsured children are more than five times more likely than the insured to have at least one unmet medical need each year, are three times less likely to get a needed prescription, and are 70 percent more likely to go without needed medical care for childhood conditions such as sore throats, ear infections, and asthma (Alliance for Health Reform).

Not surprisingly, people without health insurance end up in poorer health and with earlier deaths than those with insurance. A 2003 study comparing mortality rates of the insured and uninsured in Kentucky found significant disparities. The three-year survival rate for patients with prostate cancer was 98 percent for the insured but only 83 percent for the uninsured. For patients with breast cancer, the survival rate was 91 percent for insured patients and 78 percent for those uninsured. The comparable figures for those with colorectal cancer were 71 percent and 53 percent, and for lung cancer, 23 percent and 13 percent (McDavid et al. 2003). Countless audits of records, surveys, and analyses of data sets document that people without health insurance do not receive the health care that they need. In 2002 the Institute of Medicine, a well-respected nonprofit organization of experts who advise Congress on health issues, determined that 18,000 deaths each year can be blamed on the lack of health insurance and the resulting absence of preventive services, timely diagnoses, and appropriate care (Institute of Medicine).

FREE CLINIC PATIENTS

Background Characteristics

Age

Most free health clinics see a cross-section of the low-income and working poor members of their communities. While the hippie drug clinics commonly saw patients in their teens and twenties, the neighborhood clinics routinely saw patients across the age spectrum. As the target population began to change in free clinics, it was common to see children and to see adults up to the age of sixty-five. The assumption was made that Medicaid was handling at least most of the health care needs of the very poor and that Medicare was handling at least most of the health care needs of those sixty-five and older. For this reason, most free clinics did not and still do not provide services to the Medicaid- or Medicare-covered. As programs like SCHIP have been devised to help get health care to children and teens, most free clinics no longer see many patients in this age group. Therefore, the vast majority of free clinic patients are between twenty and sixty-four.

Over the years, however, the gaps in coverage of Medicare and Medicaid have become increasingly apparent. For those with Medicare, the absence of any coverage for prescription drugs has been a profound problem. As the cost of prescription medicines has increased by leaps and bounds in the last decade, the ability to pay for medications has been put out of reach for more and more individuals. This has created a significant dilemma for free clinics. Most do not provide medical care to the Medicare-covered because the amount of services they can provide is limited and targeted to those without any access to care and because they do not receive Medicare reimbursement. Most clinics could not at all afford to provide services for those with Medicare. At the same time, however, an important part of free clinics is being responsive to particular needs in the community. The inability of those sixty-five and older to afford their medications is a clearly perceived problem in every community.

The response made by free clinics to this dilemma has been influenced largely by the resources of the clinic. Free clinics with adequate resources have found a middle ground. While they do not provide medical care for the Medicare-covered, they will provide medications for them. This has helped to address the need, but it has done so at a tremendous financial cost to the clinics. Other clinics have not had the financial wherewithal or staff support to take on this responsibility, so they have been unable to provide medications for this group. In these communities, those sixty-five and older still often have no place to go to obtain needed medications at an affordable price. The extent to which this problem will be addressed by the Medicare prescription drug benefit passed by Congress in 2004 is as yet unclear.

Gender

As clinics are developed, it has been common for them to see more female than male patients, but for the number of male patients to increase over time. This may well be related to the general propensity of women to use more health care services than men, for women to be the primary decision makers within families about health care needs and the use of services, and by the fact that most clinics provide gynecological services that may not otherwise be easily accessible for female patients.

Income

Most free clinics see patients who lack health insurance and do not have sufficient income to purchase it. While many of the very poor do receive Medicaid assistance, it is individuals and families with an income just above the very poor—the medically indigent—who are often most vulnerable. The recent welfare reform legislation and tightening of eligibility standards for Medicaid eligibility have created more people without health insurance who are in desperate need of free clinic services.

Race and Ethnicity

Most free clinic patient populations reflect the racial and ethnic composition of the community population. Free clinics do not always have complete control over the site at which they are located in the sense that many are located in buildings that have been donated to them or at which they have obtained a very favorable lease. Because many free clinic patients do not have their own means of transportation, many walk to the clinic or use public transportation. For that reason, clinics often draw patients from their surrounding neighborhoods and reflect the racial and ethnic background of these areas. Clinics that are close to public transportation routes—often city buses—can more easily draw patients from the whole community. The most dominant recent trend—found in all parts of the country and in both large cities and smaller towns—is a substantial increase in the number of Hispanic patients. This trend is consistent with recent immigration patterns to the United States.

Occupation

Because most free clinics target their services to the working poor, patients are routinely either employed full-time or part-time, in families that are supported by a full-time or part-time worker or have been temporarily displaced from the workforce due to illness, disability, or layoff. The kinds of jobs that they have reflect the jobs in America that offer low wages and few, if any, benefits or a health insurance benefit with a cost that the employee cannot afford.

For example, North Carolina free clinics see many temporary workers (many factories now hire employees through temp agencies because it is easier to dismiss these employees and the company does not have to provide benefits to temporary workers), migrant workers (who continually migrate to wherever there is work), many small factory workers such as in textile or furniture plants (where commonly there are no health benefits or health benefits only for the employee with a prohibitively high cost to cover family members), and workers in small businesses such as nursing homes. West Virginia free clinics see many restaurant workers, especially fast-food restaurant workers, which are notorious for keeping employees' hours just beneath the level that would qualify for health insurance coverage, and workers in large department stores such as Wal-Mart and K-Mart. In Washington, D.C., many free clinic patients are people who clean homes, offices, or motels, or are home health aides, security guards, drivers, parking attendants, convenience store clerks, workers in substance abuse programs, grocery store baggers, and day care workers. In Ohio, free clinics see many factory workers who cannot afford their share of a health insurance benefit, wait staff, hairdressers, service station attendants, small business workers, workers in service industries, and fast-food restaurant workers. In California, many housekeepers, wait staff, one-person business owners, artists, actors and actresses, day laborers, and blue-collar workers often seek care in free clinics. Virginia free clinics see many fast-food restaurant workers, cafeteria workers, painters, roofers, workers in small companies, seasonal workers, and yard workers. Around the country, the same pattern emerges over and over. Workers who we may see and interact with, who we depend on for products and services, and who we may look past and never really think about work full-time or part-time for a low wage and no or unaffordable health benefits.

Genuine Need for Services

Patients come to free clinics with the same type of medical problems that are presented to primary care and specialty care providers. Sometimes there is no clinically definable illness and the reassurance of the medical provider is sufficient. Sometimes patients have general medical illnesses such as upper respiratory infections or stomach problems. In larger cities, substance abuse problems and sexually transmitted infections are not uncommon. Most commonly, however, free clinic patients are suffering from chronic conditions such as diabetes, high blood pressure, and asthma. Many patients are accustomed to just "riding out" illnesses and continuing their life until they improve or get very sick. Many come to free clinics late in the course of a disease that could have been treated effectively had they only received timely care. But, all over the country, and to an increasing extent, free clinic patients need help in diagnosing, monitoring, and treating very serious chronic conditions.

Stories of free clinic patients testify to the genuine level of need not being met in our health care system.

We have a woman who came in, I had known her a little bit because she had been in a few times before this night, but she came into the clinic one night, said that she had a really bad stomach ache, and she kept rubbing her abdomen. When the provider saw her, she found out from the description of symptoms that it was more in her chest than in her abdomen, and so we did an EKG, which was abnormal. We drove her to the hospital, and she was transferred to another hospital, and she had open heart surgery the next day. She was very sick. She was just pushing through it. She had decided that this is just the way that life is, and you just keep on going. But because she came in, we were able to get an EKG and assess her symptoms with a little bit more of an objective ear. She is probably alive today because she came in that night. After she had the surgery, she called here, she was crying, and asked me to tell the provider that she knew that she wouldn't be alive without her. She is in her early forties.

One family was referred to our clinic by the child's school. They wanted him (age ten) to have his eyes examined; his eyes were shooting off in all directions. The family had no health insurance. We found a Spanish-speaking ophthalmologist who did a diagnosis. The eye problem was being exacerbated by the boy's tonsils and adenoids. So we sent him to a pediatrician. She saw him and eventually removed his tonsils and adenoids for free, and we arranged for him to receive eyeglasses at the clinic for no charge. We also were able to provide care for the rest of his family.

A gentleman had been to the free clinic when we very first started, and then he had moved out-of-town, and then he moved back. He was working at Wal-Mart, but his insurance had not yet started. He called and said he just needed some help—that he felt so bad. So I set him up with an appointment on Thursday night. His blood sugar was 596, and his blood pressure was 200 over 120. We sent him immediately to the hospital. He has been so grateful. His blood sugar is now under 200, and the last time that he came in to get his medicine, he started to cry when he told us how appreciative he is.

One of our patients, a Black female whose husband is disabled, does work but does not have insurance. As part of the screening process, our doctor ordered a routine mammogram, and it came back with a malignant cancer. We referred her to a cooperating surgeon who removed the cancer at no charge. Had that patient not come to us with something entirely different, and in the process of seeing her, the doctor recommending a mammogram, she would likely not be alive today.

We have had two women with breast lumps that they had let go, and by the time they got here, there was little that could be done. They put it off because they were afraid of the expense. We had a young woman in her early twenties who came to us with a severe heart problem. The doctor guessed that she would have lived no more than a month. He got her into surgery immediately. She is fine now. We have had patients with chest pain and pain radiating up and down their arm who won't seek care because they are so afraid of the cost. That is very sad.

Recently, a lady called in and said that two months ago she fell, and she thinks that she dislocated her shoulder. When she comes in, the doctor determines that she had actually had a stroke. She was recently divorced, her husband was not paying alimony, she was living with her daughter, and she had not been taking her high blood pressure medicine or her diabetes medicine for over two years. We worked closely with her to address her whole situation and to get things turned around.

We have worked with a couple, both of whom are diabetic. They could not afford to purchase all of the medications that were needed. It was obvious when they came to us that they had not been taking their medicine. They even told us that they were sharing their insulin, one taking it one day and the other the next. They thought that was a little bit better than not taking any. They were struggling to do what they should do, but there were so many other issues going on in their lives. They had a hard time believing that they should spend the money to get well—they just couldn't deal with one more thing.

Recently, a gentleman came to us with some vague symptoms, but he was obviously very ill. He had been to the Department of Social Services and had tried to get a medical card and had tried to get Social Security but had failed. He probably just did not know the system well enough to know what procedures to go through. Because resources were very limited, he had run out of gas on his way to the clinic and had to walk here. As we started working him up, it became obvious that he had a very serious heart problem and kidney problem in addition to other medical problems. We have worked very hard getting him referred to different specialists, getting the tests that he needed, helping him to get in con-

tact with resources for which he is eligible. When I think about this man walk-
ing to the clinic, it is unbelievable that he even made it here. He is now in the
hospital and having a cardiac catherization today. I feel like if he had not walked
through our doors initially he would never have gotten to this point. Are his
medical problems so severe that he will not be able to overcome them? I don't
know. But at least we were able to give him a chance.

I will never forget one afternoon that we were here, a fifty-one-year-old woman
came in. She had just checked herself out of the hospital within a day after a
stroke. She said that she could not afford to be in the hospital, that she had
nowhere to go, and that somebody had told her to come here. Her speech was
still slurred, she obviously needed to be in a hospital, and here she was. So we
determined to see her and to do all of the tests that we could think of that might
help. I can still see the tears streaming down her face, "Somebody is going to help
me just because I walked in the door, and they didn't even know I was coming."

We helped a woman who came into the clinic one morning. She was wheezing,
and it was not normal for her. She had been in here before, I knew that was unusual. Normally, if someone is wheezing, I would give them albuterol nebulizer
treatment and have them see a doctor. But I said to her, "You never wheeze."
She said "No, and I gave up smoking two months ago." I put her in a room and
told the doctor that there was something bad going on here. It turns out that
she had a huge lesion on her lung. Between the time that they found it and she
started her radiation, she obstructed at home, and she had an emergency. She got
immediate care, and she is alive today.

One of the first people whom we ever helped who needed hospitalization back
in the days when we were just doing symptoms was a young Hispanic woman
who spoke little or no English. One of the volunteer physicians who was an
asthma specialist happened to be working that evening and examined her. She
complained of bronchitis. But, in examining her, he didn't like the way that the
nodes in her neck felt. So, in addition to treating, he said he would like to send
her over to the hospital to have another test done. We did the blood test, hand
carried it over to the hospital after clinic that night, and the report came back
that she had cancer. We tried to track her down and couldn't. Meanwhile, the
volunteer physician called in to check on things, and he got in his car and
tracked this woman down to tell her the result. What do we do? At that point,
we did not have a mechanism to get her admitted to the hospital or to get her
chemotherapy. The other alternative was to have her declared an illegal alien
and have her deported back to Mexico, because as it turned out, she was also
pregnant. That volunteer physician is the one who made it happen. He arranged
for her treatment in the hospital and to get the chemo she needed at no charge.
He saved her life and saved the baby.

Often, people come in with symptoms that have to do with a minor problem but
not the most serious problem. One man thought he had some respiratory illness, but we did a number of tests and determined that it might be his heart. We

set up an EKG. Before he could even get to that test, he came back in, and he was literally gray. We called the cardiologist, who sent him to the hospital and had him admitted. He had bypass surgery at no cost. While they were doing the bypass surgery, they discovered that he had a mass on his kidney that turned out to be cancerous. So we made arrangements for his care in his house until he recovered enough from the bypass surgery to have his kidney removed. And, the last we heard, he was working again at a job with health care benefits.

4

The Second Transformation in Free Health Clinics: The Shift to the Medical Mainsteam

Quietly, free clinics have been inching their way into community health care systems, and communities have found that free clinics play a major role for a segment of the population that really cannot access traditional health care due to a lack of resources.

(Estelle Nichols Avner, Executive Director, Bradley Free Clinic, Roanoke, Virginia)

THE EARLY YEARS

We have had excellent support from physicians, nurses, dentists, and other providers. Free clinics provide them a very natural and easy way to meet the code of ethics of their profession that typically includes something about giving back and giving freely of your services to people in need. Initially, I think the legislative and policy community didn't know who we were, but now that we are working with them more closely, they see the great work that we are doing and our cost-effectiveness, and, from a bottom-line perspective, what a good investment we are. Some free clinics have been started by public health directors and/or staff who saw public health moving away from providing direct services and wanted to do something to fill in the gaps—often they champion the free clinic. On the other hand, we have seen some public health directors or staffs look warily upon free clinics and be concerned about duplication of efforts, although that rarely exists. Free Clinics cannot afford to duplicate services. . . . Support from the community at large, which is critical to the success of free clinics can be measured in a number of ways. One way is to look at United Way support, and free clinics typically do very well with United Way support. There are very few naysayers. Overall, the response has been very good. (Mark Cruise, Executive Director, Virginia Association of Free Clinics)

Almost without exception, free health clinics established in the late 1960s and early 1970s in the United States were created as an alternative to the mainstream medical care system. The hippie drug clinics were based on the failure of mainstream medicine to provide adequate primary and specialty medical services to young, disaffected persons. Often, health care professionals and facilities failed to provide care in an emotionally supportive, nonjudgmental manner and failed to protect patient confidentiality. Individuals seeking care for drug-related problems, for problem pregnancies, for sexually transmitted infections, and for contraceptive services could not find available services and often felt mistreated when they did enter the medical system. The cultural chasm between the medical establishment and the mostly young people in their teens and twenties was huge and resulted in many persons failing to obtain needed medical services.

The neighborhood minority clinics were based on the failure of mainstream medicine to provide adequate primary and specialty medical services to racial and ethnic minority group members. Private medical services were often out of reach financially to low-income members of these groups, public programs offered far too few services to meet the need, and medical providers often had little training and little experience in interacting with members of other groups and sometimes little interest. A significant cultural chasm also existed between racial and ethnic minorities and white medical providers.

Early clinic organizers, whatever their personal background, typically sought to create medical services that would offer an alternative approach. They would be "free" in terms of providing care at no charge but also free in terms of eliminating extensive paperwork, intrusive means tests, and condescending and insulting judgmental attitudes. They were intentionally created to be different than the medical mainstream and not at all a part of it. They were frequently housed in storefronts or church basements rather than in expensive, glitzy buildings. Equipment and supplies were almost always donated and rarely the most modern available. Staff members including physicians often wore street clothes rather than more formal medical attire and often had patients call them by their first names. There was a de-emphasis on eligibility requirements and a clear focus on medical need. Patients who were worried about confidentiality, sometimes due to previous personal experiences, were freely permitted to use a false name. Frank discussions about lifestyle choices often occurred but in a nonjudgmental manner. There was little mainstream about the early free clinics.

The first step in getting medical care to those being left out of the system was to convince them that an alternative existed. The types of buildings in which free clinics were located may have been based largely on what was donated to them or what was the most affordable, but they made an important statement in their difference from hospitals and private physician offices. The informality—and sometimes ordered chaos—made the clinics more rather than less approachable. The fact that those providing services were typically volunteers communicated that they wanted to be treating this patient population. The assurances of confidentiality and the absence of identity and insurance checks conveyed that these were places to be trusted.

THE SHIFT TO THE MEDICAL MAINSTREAM

The second important transformation in free health clinics is that they have evolved from this "alternative" identity to becoming part of a community's mainstream medical care. Today, staff and volunteers at most free clinics consider their clinic to be an important part of the local medical care system and consider it important to be integrated within the maze of medical and social services within the community. To be sure, some free clinics have more desire than others to be part of the medical mainstream, and some are more integrated into their community's overall care system. The view of local medical professionals is not the same for all free clinics. But the dominant pattern today is that free clinics are an integral part of medical resources in the communities in which they are located.

Why this change? Why have clinics evolved from an emphasis on being an alternative to mainstream medicine to becoming part of it? There are at least four reasons to help explain this shift.

Change in Patient Population

First, and perhaps most obviously, the shift in targeted population described in chapter 3 toward the uninsured and working poor has increased the desire of free clinics to work closely with other community agencies in providing care. When clinics focused on young patients and minority patients who felt distanced from mainstream medicine, it was very important to emphasize their differences with the way medical care was routinely practiced. The manifest ways that clinics differed—nature of the building, lack of formality, emphasis on confidentiality and nonjudgmental attitudes—were necessary to get the primary intended patient population to notice the clinic and to have sufficient trust in the clinic to seek medical attention.

As the primary patient population has shifted to the uninsured and working poor, the need to be different has been replaced by an emphasis on making the provision of care be similar (in most respects) to the care offered in private physicians' offices and medical clinics. The goal now is to prevent free clinic patients from feeling that they are receiving care in substandard facilities or with substandard equipment. While the size and quality of free clinic buildings vary enormously, many are now located in new and modern facilities, and few are located in church basements. Thus, what was once important to attract patients is no longer necessary, and what was once relatively unimportant is now seen as being considerate of patients.

Three qualifications to this first reason need to be made. As mentioned earlier, a focus on the uninsured and working poor is not the only or even the primary focus in all clinics. In many large urban areas, there is still profound need for services for young persons (including drug treatment and drug rehabilitation services), for homeless persons, and for newly arrived immigrants (especially those who are undocumented). Second, while many free clinics now exist in modern facilities, there is considerable nostalgia among many staff and volunteers from the early years about the special ambience that existed in the storefronts, old houses, and church basements. While the lack of patient privacy, outmoded medical equipment, and inadequate dispensaries were hardly in patients' best interest, there was a very special atmosphere of camaraderie and closeness that often existed in the early facilities. Third, and most importantly, the shift toward the medical mainstream should not be interpreted to mean that the commitment to treating all patients with dignity and respect has been sacrificed. Volunteers at free clinics invariably still see the clinic as being a very special place that offers very special care. Many staff, volunteers, and patients express that the care offered in free clinics is in some respects (such as the amount of time given to each patient and the caring atmosphere within the clinic) superior to that often offered in private care facilities.

> The thing about free clinics is that it is people coming together—all their different gifts and talents—in a way that you can't do in other places. That is what makes free clinics so special. And I think it is still the driving force—the commitment to the core absolutely remains, and we must be sure to keep that special spirit even in new buildings. (Sheri Wood, Executive Director, Kansas City Free Health Clinic, Kansas City, Missouri)

Best Interest of Patients

Most free clinics have determined that, at this time, they can offer the best possible services to their patients by being a fully participating member of a community's medical care system and working with other medical and social service agencies. Certainly, in the early generation of free clinics, support of all kinds was received from medical providers in the community, but the extent of this support varied widely. While some free clinics secured quick support in their community, many others found that their alternative image was off-putting to other community health agents.

This created a dilemma for the free clinics. At the same time that they were criticizing the medical mainstream and consciously trying to offer medical care in an alternative way, they were dependent on support from at least some members of it. While early clinics attracted many very dedicated physicians as volunteers, difficulty obtaining an adequate number of volunteer health care providers was often a significant issue. Commonly, early free clinics were operated on shoestring budgets and depended on providers to donate equipment, supplies, and medications (often in the form of drug samples provided to physicians by pharmaceutical companies). Although the number of extremely expensive diagnostic tests and medical treatments has skyrocketed in the last forty years, obtaining these procedures for patients was a problem early on. Even four decades ago, it was difficult to provide all of the medications needed by patients. Many clinics found that the most surprising aspect of starting a free clinic was the huge need for patient medications. Clinics asked themselves what good it was to examine a patient and determine an expensive diagnostic test was needed only to be unable to secure that test and what good it was to determine that a patient required medication that the patient could not afford and the clinic could not provide.

Free clinics have acquired a rather remarkable reputation in many communities for their focus and their drive on providing the best possible medical care for their patients. Over the years, most free clinics—though not all—have determined that optimal care can be provided when there are more funds available, when more providers are willing to volunteer, when governments and foundations are more willing to sponsor needed programs, and when there is a more integrated effort with other community services to assist patients. Did this lead to an identifiable pivotal point within each clinic's history at which it decided to be less alternative and more mainstream? No. Clinic directors can remember no such identifiable point nor even any obvious discussion threads about making such a transition. Rather, the shift to being an integral part of a community's medical resources evolved over time within clinics. It occurred as society changed from the activist counterculture of the 1960s and early 1970s. It occurred as communities increasingly recognized the high quality of care provided in free clinics. It occurred as both the cost of private medical care and the number of people without insurance escalated. It occurred when clinic directors spoke to medical societies and church groups and local governments and civic groups, and more people in the communities recognized the valuable service being provided.

> I think free clinics need to be part of the system, not an alternative to it. To say they are an alternative, to me, has the connotation of being not as good as. So I would say we should be part of the system. The physicians who come here say over and over that this is what they went to school for, this is how they want to practice medicine, and that here they can focus on their patients. They don't have to worry about whether or not an insurance policy will allow them to

order a test. They can come in, they can see their patients, they can order tests that they need, they can get the lab work they need, and they do not have to worry about filing insurance forms. In a way, patients here are getting better care than if they were insured and getting care in a physician's office, because insurance often dictates that unless you have a particular symptom, then you can't test for a particular disease until much later. If the doctors here want to look for something, they can do it. You don't have to wait until three months down the road when the patient develops additional symptoms. (Carla Bice, St. Joseph Health Center, South Bend, Indiana)

Support from local hospitals has long been extremely important in the ability of free clinics to offer their patients access to expensive diagnostic tests. Almost every free clinic has established a relationship with one or more hospitals in which the hospital provides diagnostic procedures to free clinic patients at no charge (in some cases, at reduced charge) and analyzes laboratory tests that have been done on-site at the clinic. Some free clinics also benefit from free testing donated by private diagnostic laboratories. Whatever size their budget, free clinics are simply not able to pay for expensive hospital tests and procedures for all of their patients who desperately need them.

In South Bend, Indiana, the local hospital does testing, x-rays, even surgeries for free clinic patients at no charge, and the anesthesiologists and radiologists do not charge for their services. A private laboratory does all of the lab work for free. In Columbia, Maryland, Quest Diagnostics does all of the blood work for free clinic patients at no charge; Advanced Radiology provides all radiological services at no charge; Open MRI provides all magnetic resonance imaging tests at no charge. In community after community, in-kind support from hospitals, and though less regularly, from private diagnostic laboratories, is an important part of the effectiveness of free clinics and significantly widens the range of services available to free clinic patients.

In Lakewood [Ohio], we have three local hospitals: Lakewood Hospital, Fairview Park Hospital, and St. John Westshore Hospital. Our first executive director and first physician went to each of the hospitals and made a strong case for donating services to free clinic patients. Today, they donate direct clinical services, hospitalization, and testing. This is all about relationships. Our abiding principle is that we do not duplicate services. (Lee Elmore, Executive Director, North Coast Health Ministry, Lakewood, Ohio)

Our free clinic has been a collaborative effort since the beginning. The local hospital has been a major supporter of the clinic, not in dollars, but in doing all of our lab work, all of our diagnostic procedures, even some surgery for clinic patients with no charge. Last year, they provided more than $90,000 in free care. (Sandy Motley, Davidson Medical Ministries Clinic, Inc., Lexington, North Carolina)

From the standpoint of physicians, an available free clinic is a great service to have because it gives them someplace to send people. I think most physicians feel frustrated when they have to say, "I don't know what to do for you." It is such an overwhelming problem. Private practice offices can only do so much free care or they stop being able to pay the rent. The biggest problem that I can see has always been on the higher end of things. What do I do with the free clinic patient who has cancer, or the free clinic patient who needs an MRI, or who needs epidural injections, or who has a chronic problem with complications, and I have a $3,000 budget. One MRI is $2,000. The only way that you can exist is to have someone give you the service for free, because even 25 percent or 50 percent or 75 percent off would bleed your funds. (Tom Rives, MD, Friendship House, Conway, South Carolina)

Increased Stability of Clinics

Inextricably linked with the best interest of patients is the third reason for this transition: increased stability for the free clinics themselves. The creation of free clinics in the late 1960s and early 1970s made a profound statement. Community activists, including many medical providers, took on the responsibility of providing needed medical services that were not being offered or were not being offered well by the medical mainstream. Imagine the disparity in access to funds between a private medical clinic that accepts private and public health insurance dollars and a free clinic just getting started in a donated building with donated equipment and supplies and a mostly volunteer staff. The fact that some of these early free clinics, like the Haight-Ashbury Free Clinics, the Berkeley Free Clinic, the Washington Free Clinic, the Fan Free Clinic (Richmond, VA), the Kansas City Free Health Clinic, and the Free Clinic of Greater Cleveland, have survived for thirty or more years and continue to grow and offer services is a remarkable testimony to the dedication of the early and present-day staff and volunteers. But many more of the early free clinics have not survived.

While becoming more of a part of the medical mainstream cannot be said to have been essential in surviving (the Berkeley Free Clinic being an example of a clinic that continues to cherish its alternative basis), most of the clinics that survived—and almost none of those that did not—have done so in part by becoming a more integral and integrated part of the local medical system. The specific channels through which free clinics have benefited include: expanded lists of individual and corporate financial support; financial support from local and state governments, private foundations, and community fund-raising groups such as United Way; more volunteers; significant contributions of in-kind (and sometimes financial) support from local hospitals; cooperative relationships with public health departments; and vast networking arrangements with community and social service agencies.

Greater Contributions to the Health Care System

As free clinics have developed more extensive ties within community health care systems, there has been increased opportunity to provide benefits to the system itself. Two of the most important ways that this occurs are through providing educational experiences for undergraduate, graduate, and health professional students and through contributions to health policy formulation at the local, state, and national levels.

Almost all of the free clinics in communities with a college or university provide internship and volunteer opportunities for undergraduate and graduate students. While these students may come from almost any academic field, many of them are studying premed, prenursing, prepharmacy, physical or occupational therapy, nutrition, or other areas in the health field. Many are social science majors who anticipate working in the health sector with their undergraduate or graduate degree. Many medical schools located in a community with a free clinic encourage their students to volunteer at the clinic, and many medical residents give volunteer hours to a local clinic.

These experiences can be real eye-openers. For many students, it is their first real opportunity to work with patients who lack the financial wherewithal to afford private medical care. They may encounter social situations that impact on health or medical conditions that they have not worked with personally. It may be the first exposure to community medicine. At the same time as they are learning from their experience, they are providing a valuable service to the patients. Whether the student is conducting a personal or medical history, counting pills from samples in the pharmacy, or, in the case of residents, providing clinical services, the patients and clinic benefit from their efforts. In addition, many physicians who volunteered at a free clinic during their residency become committed volunteers at a free clinic in the community where they ultimately locate and become strong advocates for free clinics.

> We have found that one of the functions that free clinics serve is providing training in community medicine for doctors and health officials. Often, these individuals then move on into the medical care system, and they have taken some of these ideals and concepts with them. You think now of hospitals that make beds available to indigent patients. That did not exist before free clinics. It is really not that apparent until you look closely at what has happened and see these effects. (Richard Seymour, Director of Training and Education, Haight-Ashbury Free Clinics, San Francisco, California)

In addition free clinic staff are playing an increasing role in community discussions of general and particular health care needs, the location of proposed health care services, and the amount of public and private funds that should be allocated to health needs in general or to a free clinic in particular. Studies of community power structures routinely find that a network of individuals circulates through key decision-making positions. They may serve on the board of directors of corporations, banks, and hospitals and also on the boards of community social service agencies and civic groups. Especially in small and medium-sized communities, these individuals usually know each other, may interact socially as well as professionally, and have an enormous impact on decisions that affect the community. For free clinic staff, the question often is simply whether it is better to be part of this network or not. When the best interests of the free clinic and the best interests of free clinic patients are considered, more and more free clinic directors, other staff, and volunteers are opting to participate.

The voice of free clinic people also is increasingly being heard at the state level and even at the national level. Several free clinic directors have testified before state government committees on health-related matters. Kevin Kelleher, MD, a twenty-year-plus volunteer (including serving as medical director) at the Bradley Free Clinic in Roanoke, Virginia, has become a key national spokesperson for free clinics. He was one of just a few individuals who testified before Congress and helped to get passed the Volunteer Protection Act, legislation that helps protect volunteers from legal liability suits. During the Clinton Administration, Kelleher served on the Task Force on Charitable Care and advised it on ways that free clinics could contribute to unmet health care needs in the country. He has published several articles on free clinics and is frequently called upon to share his expertise. The final chapter in this book examines the future for free clinics and revisits ways in which free clinics are contributing to the national health care policy discussion.

I think free health clinics have become an integral part of the system. Here in Kansas City, we are at the table with community health centers, the public hospital, and others. Free clinics need the support of the community. The reason that the county hospital and the city are so supportive of us is that we can see a patient for far less than they can be seen someplace else in the community because of our use of volunteers. I also understand that the continuity of care here is less than in the community, so we are hoping to give referrals for patients beyond our scope. We are a teaching site for all of the hospitals around here. One of the community health agencies sends their midwife to us to provide programs. We really believe in collaboration. We work with African-American churches and with alternative schools to provide programming. Free clinics can be a real force in the community. It is the only way to make it work. We really believe "you talk it, you walk it." It is not the easiest way to provide care; it has its frustrations, but it is what we need to do. (Sheri Wood, Executive Director, Kansas City Free Health Clinic, Kansas City, Missouri)

My idealistic view is to say that we are part of the health care system. We are seen as a safety net clinic. It may be that some see us as separate—as just a bunch of do-gooders who are trying to help and that there are other alternatives for these patients. I think the idea that the government is going to pick up where private insurance leaves off is unfortunate thinking. It is not true. Finally, people are starting to recognize free health clinics as being part of the medical care system. In the Chicago area we constantly fight to be part of the community planning process. For example, a recent community needs assessment concluded that the city needs another health clinic—right here. We asked, "Why didn't you address us?" The answer was, "Well, we knew you were there but . . . " We have 16,000 patient visits per year. Does the city want them all in the emergency room? (Laura Michalski, Director of Clinical Relations, CommunityHealth, Chicago, Illinois)

COMMUNITY RECEPTIVITY TO FREE HEALTH CLINICS

The benefits of community integration of free clinics to the clinics account for only part of the high level of acceptance and considerable support that have been gained from other medical providers. After all, in the United States, the medical marketplace is fiercely competitive: hospitals compete with other hospitals and physicians compete with each other for patients; insurance companies compete to sell health policies; and public (for example, public health departments) and private health agencies compete for dollars from governments, foundations, and private donors. Free clinics are created within this competitive arena and must rely on support from others in the arena for their success.

Four reasons are most important in explaining the remarkable support typically won by free clinics: community-wide perception that a significant problem exists, a belief in the effectiveness of free clinics in helping to meet this problem, an understanding that the free clinic will not duplicate services provided by others, and recognition that the free clinic will facilitate more efficient use of hospital resources by reducing use of emergency rooms for nonemergency visits.

Community-Wide Perception of Problem

Arguably, the most important prerequisite for the support given to free clinics is a perception that inadequate access to health care services for some groups is a significant problem in the community. Most clinic directors have found overwhelming recognition of this problem in their community. Studies conducted in the United States routinely show that the high cost of health care and inadequate access to health care are perceived as being among the most serious national problems. Community-wide needs assessments (studies done within communities to identify the most serious "needs" of local people) almost always pinpoint access to health care as the most serious or one of the most serious needs. Even individuals and families with health insurance often are concerned about its limitations, and many people justifiably fear that a serious medical crisis within the family would leave them in financial ruins. In some ways, the nation's uninsured and underinsured are invisible: one can't determine a person's insurance status just by looking at him or her, and it is difficult to feel the suffering that might be experienced by another who cannot get needed medical attention or afford prescribed medications. But there is at least a general sense that a significant social problem exists.

The experience of the second generation of free clinics—those started in the 1980s, 1990s, and since the turn of the century—attests to this understanding of the problem. Almost none of these clinics faced any significant opposition in getting started, and most experienced no opposition at all.

> I have not personally faced any opposition to the clinic. I am waiting for that day when I give a speech, and somebody comes up to me afterwards and says that those people ought to pull themselves up by their bootstraps and take care of their own problems. I intend to respond, "Well, that would be nice if saying that made it work, but, it doesn't!" (Parker Sparrow, Executive Director, Free Medical Clinic, Columbia, South Carolina)

Effectiveness of Free Health Clinics in Addressing the Problem

Second, the success of free clinics in becoming integrated into the community is based on having convinced the community of the quality of medical services that are provided. Even though the quality of care provided in the early free clinics was often very high, some individuals still have the mental image of a free clinic as a MASH unit, and they must be persuaded that is not the case. Free clinics have used many strategies to overcome this misperception. Probably the most important effort has been to create an environment in which quality medical care is practiced. This has typically been accomplished by having a health care professional—usually a physician but possibly a nurse or nurse practitioner—who serves as the medical director of the clinic. This individual may or may not be a paid staff member, but it is someone who accepts responsibility for ensuring that the medical care actually being delivered is of high standards. This facet also has important symbolic value, as it increases the trust level of other community health care professionals in the quality of the medical service being provided.

Free clinics have employed other strategies as well: invitations to key individuals for guided tours of the clinic, written testimonies from health care professionals, and, most importantly, word of mouth. Without exception, free clinics have found that word-of-mouth contacts by current physician-volunteers are the most effective way to attract new volunteers. Many people are constantly solicited by requests for financial or in-kind support for worthy causes. No one can respond affirmatively to all of the requests, but the most effective way to solicit help or a contribution is through direct personal contact with individuals in one's social or professional network. This enables the recruiter to target those whose values would support free clinics and free clinic participation, and it carries the extra persuasiveness of personal appeal (Klandermans and Oegema 1987; Snow, Zurcher, and Ekland-Olson 1980). This strategy also applies to spreading the general reputation of the clinic as well. Individuals who volunteer at a free clinic are in the best position to tell their colleagues about the quality of its service.

> Particularly with licensed providers, we have found that the best recruiters are other providers. We can go to medical meetings and put articles in newsletters and get nothing. But, if a physician or nurse practitioner speaks to one of their peers and says, "This is what I do, come join me," the success rate is much higher. (James Beckner, Fan Free Clinic, Richmond, Virginia)

> Our initial board of directors went out with Dr. Sloughman almost handpicking people in the community asking if they would come on board and support this cause. There was a huge telephone campaign that was done at the end of 1991 just before the clinic opened for the construction campaign. We raised $200,000 to do the renovation of the building, but we had such wonderful response from the community—for example, Habitat got on board to provide labor, local contractors got on board—that we ended up spending less than 10 percent of what we had raised. So the community, just by word of mouth and messages through the churches and the local newspaper, got involved. We don't have a local television station, and we don't have access to a lot of media sources that other cities and urban areas would have. So it truly has been a grassroots, word-of-mouth, one-person-telling-another effort. (Sandy Motley, Executive Director, Davidson Medical Ministries Clinic, Inc., Lexington, North Carolina)

> As far as physician volunteers, we try to have personal recruitment. We try to have physicians recruit physicians. When a new physician comes into their practice, comes into the community, when they have their meetings at the hospitals, they will plead the case that we need volunteers. The interesting thing is that when these new young physicians hear about us, they are really anxious to come. It is a different population. Most of them have been raised with parents who have done some kind of volunteer work, and that has been a lifestyle for them, so they are ready to come in to volunteer. The same thing is true with nurses and pharmacists—they pretty much recruit their own. Just at the last clinic that we had, we called the volunteers to remind them to come, and the pharmacist said his pharmacy tech is interested, would we mind if he brought her along. So she came that night. When I go into the community to speak—last Saturday, I spoke to the United Methodist women—I usually put in a plug for us and ask them to ask their doctor if he or she volunteers here, and then to thank them or encourage them to do so. I tell them that if they have friends who are nurses, if they know someone who is interested in doing clerical things, to refer them to us. Also, we have a group in town called Volunteer Action, and

when we need a volunteer quickly, we can call them and tell them about our particular need. They will run an ad in the newspaper for us at no charge. They will get applications from people, narrow them down, and then call me. We have gotten excellent volunteers from them. (Cynthia Moore, Clinic Director, Good Samaritan Clinic, Parkersburg, West Virginia)

In addition to the quality of care that is provided, many free health clinics are recognized in their communities for being able to bring together at one site a wide range of medical and social services. Free clinic primary care physicians often can refer patients to specialists who also volunteer at the clinic. Many of the clinics have established nonmedical social service programs and are able to connect patients with other needed services. Clinic staff and volunteers understand that if they see a need, they are encouraged to find ways for the clinic to meet the need or ways to facilitate connecting patients to available services in the community. Many clinics now offer special chronic disease programs because so many of their patients have hypertension, diabetes, and other chronic conditions. The need for free dental care is pervasive in communities, and many free clinics have established dental programs.

As examples, the Venice Family Clinic in California offers prenatal care programs; adult and pediatric services; chronic disease care for hypertensives, diabetics, and patients with heart disease and asthma; a women's health care program (including well-woman services and breast and cervical cancer screening); an HIV program; mental health counseling, health education, and medications. In addition to basic primary care services, the Canton (Ohio) Community Clinic provides services in dentistry, chiropractic, massage therapy, mental health counseling, substance abuse counseling, nutrition counseling, eye care (by ophthalmologists and optometrists), and medications. The Kalamazoo (Michigan) Free Clinic offers primary care services, eye care, dental services (through referral), medications, and a behavioral health program. The Bradley Free Clinic (Virginia) provides primary care and dental care and eight subspecialty care services including programs in rheumatology, ophthalmology, psychiatry, and plastic surgery. At Christmas, children are able to select from donated gifts in order to have something to give to family members. The Washington, D.C., Free Clinic offers four major clinical services: general medicine and family planning, HIV, prenatal care, and pediatric care. The Hollywood (California) Sunset Free Clinic includes a food and clothes pantry, a mobile unit for screening homeless patients, a Thanksgiving luncheon, and a children's Christmas party. They go to schools to do free health checkups and provide a free tattoo removal program (former gang members can get a tattoo removed in exchange for thirty volunteer hours). Americares Free Clinics in Connecticut has purchased a mobile medical unit (thanks to a $100,000 gift specifically for it) because that was determined to be helpful in making care access easier for patients and providers;

in addition to a wide range of primary and specialty care services, the Los Angeles Free Clinic maintains public showers because they are needed by the area homeless.

Some of the specialty care efforts have been developed into full-scale health education programs. The following describes diabetes education programming in one free clinic.

> There were multiple diabetes education programs carried out in the clinic setting. These were planned and implemented by graduate students in the community nutrition and health education programs at a local university. One of the diabetes education programs consisted of five sessions offered once per week over consecutive weeks. Each session focused on a different topic, such as the food guide pyramid, and included meal planning activities. Blood glucose, body weight, and blood pressure were checked and recorded at each meeting. Each week, participants were given handouts to reinforce the general concepts discussed during the class session. The point of the sessions was to provide basic nutrition information related to managing diabetes with hands-on interactive activities to apply the information to daily living. Attendance at the sessions was voluntary, but all were well-attended, indicating the patients' desire for health promotion and disease prevention services. Informal reports from patients and clinicians indicate positive effects for those patients participating in the intervention. The patients especially liked activity portions of the sessions, and many said it helped them remember the information better than just hearing it from the doctor or nurse. (Bibeau et al. 1997, 88)

Almost all free clinics now have a pharmaceutical program that enables their patients to receive most or all of their medications for free or token payment. Given the very high price of drugs, how is it possible for these volunteer-driven clinics collectively to provide millions of dollars of medications each year? The answer is that they use every legitimate means available to obtain drugs for dispensing, including (1) use of drug samples; (2) special discount arrangements with local pharmacies; (3) applications to the indigent medication program sponsored by many pharmaceutical companies; and (4), when all else fails, direct purchase of drugs.

First, many physicians and pharmaceutical representatives donate pill samples to free clinics. Often, these are one pill per package (or one pill per package compartment), and they must be removed, organized, and grouped in order to be available for the clinic pharmacist to dispense. This is a very slow and methodical process. A common sight at free clinics is that of volunteers sitting at large tables processing these drug samples. They do so because these drugs do not cost the clinic anything, and they can be made available to patients at no charge.

Second, some clinics have entered into special arrangements with local pharmacies to receive drugs for their patients at reduced (usually) or no charge. The pharmacies do this as a public service and count on the free clinic to ensure that the patient genuinely needs the medication and that a physician has written the prescription. Sometimes this works through a voucher system and sometimes the clinic obtains the medication to dispense.

Third, many of the large pharmaceutical companies sponsor indigent medication programs. In order to secure medications in this way, a free clinic staff or volunteer completes the lengthy paperwork and sends it to the appropriate pharmaceutical company. If everything is in order, the pharmaceutical company sends a supply of the medication to the free clinic to dispense to the patient. Other agents could assist low-income patients with this process, but few do because it occupies so many hours. Free clinics have taken on the chore. Finally, when medications cannot be obtained any other way, free clinics will spend what money they can to purchase the needed drugs. Given the high cost of medications and given that most free clinics rely on private donations, there are limits to how much can be purchased. The cost of purchasing drugs is a major budget component for many free clinics.

Do all of these efforts add up to a significant contribution to patients? Almost beyond belief. St. Joseph Health Center (South Bend, Indiana) fills more than one hundred prescriptions *each day*. The Will-Grundy Medical Center (Joliet, Illinois) provides more than $300,000 in medications annually; the Free Clinic of Reidsville and Vicinity, Inc. (North Carolina), provides over $250,000 in medications to patients each year; the Crisis Control Ministry (Winston-Salem, North Carolina) provides $1.4 million in medications each year; the Free Medical Clinic (Columbia, South Carolina) provides $700,000 in medications annually; $800,000 in annual medications is provided by the Kalamazoo (Michigan) Free Clinic. In Virginia, every dollar spent by free clinics on drugs is leveraged (through samples, discounts, and the indigent medication program) to seven dollars in medications that go to patients.

Nonduplication of Services

In most communities, it has been extremely important for the free clinic to demonstrate that it does not duplicate services provided by others. Certainly, it is important to the clinic not to duplicate. Needs are so great that it would be unfortunate to focus time, effort, and money on services already being provided to the target population. From the point of view of other providers, there is a natural reluctance to contribute to or volunteer at a facility that is not adding anything to the array of already existing services.

The most logical potential overlap exists with local public health departments. These departments are funded by the government to serve the public health needs of communities. However, the services provided by public health departments can differ enormously from state to state and sometimes even within states. Some departments offer direct patient services, but some do not. Many offer special programs in areas such as HIV testing, but not all do. Some offer free dental care, but most don't. Few offer services in evening hours when it would be maximally convenient for most employed persons to attend.

In many areas public health department staff, recognizing that more health care service provision is needed, have been early and strong supporters of free clinics. But, typically, they have wanted to be assured that the free clinic was not going to duplicate health department services and become a competitor for public support and public dollars. In a few cases, support from the local public health department has been less forthcoming based on a concern about potential overlap.

So most free clinics have been very careful not to duplicate services. If the local public health department offers, for example, basic physical exams required for participating in athletics in school, then the free clinic will not. If the public health department does not offer these exams, then the free clinic might, because children of the working poor might not be able to participate otherwise. If a local public health department offers eye care, the free clinic will not. But it might offer eye care if the clinic would be the only available area provider for some individuals.

Thus, what could conceivably be a contentious relationship is usually one of mutual support. The public health department in Kansas City, Missouri, for example, donated materials (for example, gowns, physicians' stools, and bandages) to the free clinic as it was getting started. When the Will-Grundy Medical Center in Joliet, Illinois, was getting started, the local public health department did not offer primary health care services and was very supportive of the free clinic. Later, when the health department added its own primary care clinic, attention was given to a possible duplication of services. When it was assured that duplicative services would not be offered, its support for the clinic continued. In Racine, Wisconsin, the free clinic and the health department are careful not to duplicate services, and they provide ongoing patient referrals to each other. The Charlottesville (Virginia) Free Clinic is located in a building actually owned by and shared by the health department; rent-free space is provided for the free clinic. The Free Medical Clinic of Northern Shenandoah Valley (Winchester, Virginia) runs a dental program in collaboration with the health department.

> We have always ensured that the programs of the health department and our programs do not duplicate. We work with them collaboratively in women's health, tuberculosis screening, sexually transmitted diseases, and other areas. They do school physicals and immunizations, but we help out in August when things get really tight. But we have limited resources, and they have limited resources, and it works like a marriage to maximize what we each have available. (Linda Cornelius, Executive Director, Augusta Regional Free Clinic, Fishersville, Virginia)

There is a second way that the issue of nonduplication of services occurs, and it relates to an important philosophical difference among free clinics. The issue pertains to having eligibility requirements to be seen at the clinic. Many clinics—especially those that were created in the early years—strongly believe that free clinics ought to be available to anyone who seeks services from them. They believe that there may be many reasons that a person would go to a free clinic. Lack of financial wherewithal to pay for private care is an obvious reason, but it might be due to feeling mistreated in the private care system or feeling more comfortable with the staff and volunteers at a free clinic or seeking a specific kind of care offered at a free clinic. Some clinics believe that all of these reasons and others are understandable and that no one should be turned away from a medical care site. For these clinics, part of what it means to be "free" is, when you are sick, to be free of eligibility requirements, means tests, and questions about personal finances.

For example, the Free Clinic of Greater Cleveland is willing to treat anyone who comes to the clinic but counsels those who could access private care to do so. The clinic explains that this is done to try to ensure that the free clinic services that are available get to individuals without other care options. The Fan Free Clinic in Richmond, Virginia, continues to function without eligibility requirements; services are open to anyone who requests them as long as there are space and services available.

Other free clinics—especially those created since 1980—are more likely to have eligibility requirements. Typically, requirements relate to family size, family income, and having or being eligible for Medicare or Medicaid. Some clinics ask just a brief question or two, while others require physical documentation (typically, a pay check stub or tax form). Some conduct this review only the first time a patient appears at the clinic; others do it periodically. The rationale for having eligibility requirements is that they enable free clinics to target their services to those with medical needs that cannot be attended to elsewhere. If someone can afford private care or has insurance to pay for private care, then that person is referred to a private provider, and a spot is opened up for someone unable to obtain services elsewhere. Some physician volunteers at free clinics explain that they are willing to donate their time and service to patients unable to pay, but that they do not want to provide gratis services for individuals who could pay to see them or another provider.

For example, in Kansas City, Missouri, the only eligibility requirement is that the patient not have health insurance. St. Joseph Health Center in South Bend, Indiana, has only the requirements that patients be below 150 percent of the federally established poverty level and not have any form of health insurance. At CommunityHealth in Chicago, there is a one-page screening form with the key question being whether or not the individual or family has health insurance. One question is asked about income (officially, 200 percent of the poverty level is considered the cutoff, but no one is ever turned away). The clinic does not want to ask intrusive questions, so that is the priority. Davidson Medical Ministries in Lexington, North Carolina, typifies clinics with a more elaborate eligibility system.

All clients go through an eligibility process initially and periodically thereafter. They must live in this county, be uninsured, be under 200 percent of the federal poverty level, and they must provide proof of household income. They cannot have Medicare or Medicaid except for pharmacy services. We identify all of their income plus all of their expenses. We subtract the expenses from the income and subtract a buffer. If they have a negative balance, they are eligible for all of our services. If they have a positive balance, say $100, then we figure they could buy $100 worth of medicines, and the clinic will help with their other medicines. . . . If the patient is on a fixed income, we repeat the process annually. If the patient is working, we do it every six months. If the income is unstable, we ask if things have changed every time. If the patient is not insured due to unemployment, then we have a job search form, and they must be out trying to find a job. Just like at the employment commission, they must show proof of having visited three places. If the patient is living off grandma, then we check her income. We know these are tough eligibility requirements, but they are necessary in order for us to provide services to those who need them the most. We have some patients who have been here for ten years, but they are working, they do not have insurance, and they are just scraping by. (Sandy Motley, Executive Director, Davidson Medical Ministries Clinic, Inc., Lexington, North Carolina)

Efficient Use of Hospital Services

Finally, the availability of primary care services at free clinics enables many of the uninsured working poor to receive necessary care there rather than go to a hospital emergency room. Clearly, emergency room care is very expensive, and it is usually inappropriate for nonemergency purposes. But emergency rooms may be required to see anyone who goes there and may otherwise be reluctant to turn away any patients. Often, triage staff and physicians cannot determine whether a case truly requires immediate attention until an examination occurs. At that point, completing the case is more desirable than stopping in midstream. In some cases, recognizing that alternative sources of care are unavailable to a patient, hospitals provide the necessary primary care service. The perception that hospital emergency rooms are used by the uninsured as a primary care site often is accurate.

From the perspective of the patient, this is an unfortunate situation. Hospital emergency rooms are set up to provide the best possible emergency service but not necessarily the best possible primary care service. Typically, patients would be better off receiving primary care from a primary care specialist. When uninsured patients obtain primary care in an emergency room, they are charged a significantly higher rate than they would be in a physician's office or clinic setting. They may or may not anticipate paying this bill, but typically they are not able to do so. Some hospitals set up a reimbursement plan of only a few dollars a month, which provides minimal income for the hospital. For patients, it may mean carrying a large debt burden—often for the rest of their life—an embarrassing and degrading position.

> In 1994, a group of physicians and nurses at the Howard County General Hospital, the only hospital in this county, noticed that they were continually seeing in the emergency room patients with underlying illnesses such as heart disease, cancer, high blood pressure, and asthma. They recognized that if these people would be getting treatment for the underlying disease, they would not have to come to the emergency room. They were seeing people with diabetes who had not gotten any treatment and were at the point of amputation. At first, the clinic staff thought that if they could get every physician to take one patient into his or her office, the problem could be combated. Given the amount of time involved, complications that occurred, and the need for tests, it was decided that a clinic would be best, so that was created. (Pam Mack, Executive Director, Health Alliance for Patients in Need, Columbia, Maryland)

From the perspective of the health care system and the hospital, use of the emergency room for nonemergent care is very cost-inefficient. In cases in which little or no payment is made, the hospital must absorb the cost or transfer it to patients able to pay with insurance or on their own. Their bills must be increased in order to cover the unreimbursed bills. When insurance companies pay higher bills, they pass on that cost to the purchaser of the insurance, thus requiring everyone to pay more. With uncompensated care at hospitals now totalling more than $20 billion per year, this is a systemwide problem.

Any mechanism that enables uninsured patients to obtain primary care from primary care providers would be of significant benefit to patients, hospitals, and the health care system. And, that is exactly what free clinics do, and this is one of the primary arguments made to hospital directors to help justify their provision of services at no charge to free clinic patients (Nadkarni and Philbrick 2003). This makes the argument that helping free clinics is not only a humanitarian gesture but also one that is in the hospital's own financial interest. In community after community, this hypothesis has been borne out in reality. Communities around the country have detected that the free clinic provides primary care to patients who would otherwise not receive care or be forced to obtain it in a hospital emergency room.

> Soon after we opened, the Director of the Emergency Department [at the local hospital] called to say that the emergency room was an inappropriate place for the care of non-paying patients with primary care problems, and he wondered if they could refer those patients to us. I agreed that they belonged in our clinic, and we would welcome them. I then asked if we could use the emergency department as the referral point for our patients who needed secondary or tertiary

care. He agreed and the deal was struck. We have records for only the first year of operation and it appears we reduced by at least one-third the number of non-paying primary care patients who used the hospital ER. The increase in patient visits our second and third years suggests we reduced the number of non-paying patients on the ER by the same figure, suggesting we then took one-half of the remaining non-paying patients. This resulted in significant savings to the local 64-bed hospital between $650,000 and $750,000 per year. (McConnell 1998, 122–23)

When we initially went to Norwalk Hospital, they were shocked that the free clinic wanted free services. So we made the traditional argument to them about more efficient use of the emergency room. Shortly before the clinic opened, they agreed to give us a specified number of services. Since then, they have seen the benefits and have increased their quota of services to us to a very reasonable level. When we later went to Danbury Hospital, they agreed to do all of whatever we need. Both hospitals have representation on our advisory board and work closely with us. In southwestern Connecticut, neither of the two hospitals originally participated, but now one does. (Karen Gottlieb, Executive Director of Americares Free Clinics [a consortium of free clinics], based in New Canaan, Connecticut)

Hospitals typically grow very fond of free clinics . . . there may be some initial reticence, but it doesn't take long for them to recognize (1) that free clinics reduce unnecessary hospital admissions and use of the emergency room, (2) that they provide an excellent way for hospitals to utilize their charitable funds, when their mission is compatible with that, and (3) because they are truly community-based and community-built and community-supported, that free clinics very quickly become very significant organizations in the community. (Mark Cruise, Executive Director, Virginia Association of Free Clinics)

5

The Third Transformation in Free Health Clinics: The Move Toward Collective Organization

> Free clinics' greatest strength is also their Achilles Heel, and that is that we are truly community-based.
>
> (James Beckner, Fan Free Clinic)

THE EARLY YEARS

> Free clinics were not created after the general style of most official formal organizations. (Sometimes they hardly manage to maintain any organizational integrity at all.) One might better call them "free form" community medical centers. Emphasis is on adapting to the health care needs peculiar to the community in which the clinic first emerges. Emphasis is also placed on serving the needs of patients, not treating at the convenience of the bureaucracy. (Smith, Bentel, and Schwartz 1971)

Imagine what it would have been like to create a free health clinic in the late 1960s and early 1970s. You recognize that there is a significant problem in the country in that many young people feel unable to access or to trust the private health care system or you recognize that many members of racial and ethnic minority groups are unable to afford or find accessible private medical care in their community. Perhaps you have one or two allies or even a small group of activists who share your belief that this is wrong, and you all want to do something about it. You conclude that you lack the power to change the entire health care system, but you think it may be feasible to create small oases within communities that will provide care to those left out of the private care system. You are committed to the idea, and you are passionate about it. But, to start with, there is no money, no location for a clinic, no equipment, and no providers. Perhaps just as importantly, there are no models to emulate, no one with experience and expertise to offer guidance, and no manuals or literature on the subject. What a daunting task!

Yet, this is exactly the situation in which the pioneering free health clinics found themselves. In communities around the country, especially in large cities to which young people were flocking, local activists coalesced to attempt to put together a viable free medical clinic. Between 1967 and 1969, seventy free health clinics were founded in the U.S. and Canada.

While there was some interaction among free clinic people in these first few years, clinics were of necessity focused on their own day-to-day survival. Most were largely unaware of each other, and there was no easy way (in the pre-Internet days) to identify what clinics existed in what communities. The Haight-Ashbury Free Clinics, the Berkeley Free Clinic, and the Los Angeles Free Clinic were among the best-known free clinics in large part because of the visibility of the youth movement in these communities. The free clinic in the Haight-Ashbury district of San Francisco received the most national publicity, based both on the tremendous need for services in that area and on David Smith's ability to articulate the mission and philosophy of free clinics.

The fact that each of these early clinics was more or less on its own is understandable. The communities were different, the needs were different, the available resources were different, the initial spark for the clinic was different, and it was a different time. It would not have made sense to have a single model that all clinics tried to follow. But, on the other hand, the limited interaction made it difficult to share accumulated wisdom and knowledge, and the birth and maturation of these clinics were extraordinarily difficult. The early free clinics were often isolated within their own community and isolated from other free clinics, and they lacked the support that would have come from a strong network.

It is not surprising that many of these clinics survived only a short time. Several were closed by the end of the 1960s, and many more closed in the 1970s. Of these original clinics, fewer than ten still exist today.

THE RISE OF THE NATIONAL FREE CLINIC COUNCIL

As early as 1968, David Smith recognized a need for some form of central free clinic organization that could facilitate information sharing and assist with problem solving. A few clinics had begun reaching out for each other to seek advice, to compare their approaches, and to share information, and Smith hoped to build on this interest. Among his other responsibilities at this time, Smith was teaching a course on community approaches to drug abuse at the University of California–Berkeley. There, he conversed with Jim Sternfield of the Berkeley Free Clinic about common problems faced by their clinics. In

October 1968, Smith, Sternfield, Alice DeSwarte, and Carter Mehl of the Haight-Ashbury Free Clinic and several founders of the Berkeley Free Clinic met to plan a national free clinic organization (Seymour and Smith 1986).

They envisioned an organization that would be focused on education and information sharing about community needs and on educational and treatment programs that could help address those needs. The desire was to offer assistance to groups wishing to start a free clinic and to existing free clinics in resolving clinic issues and problems. They formulated organizational bylaws that divided the country into six geographic regions and included provisions to ensure adequate representation for racial and ethnic minorities, women, and gays. A twenty-five-dollar annual membership fee was created with members being provided National Free Clinic Council (NFCC) (as it was being called) publications; attendance at a psychopharmacology conference in August 1969; and attendance at a first (hopefully) annual NFCC symposium in January 1970. David Smith later recounted that "The electricity for this first meeting was high. There was a lot of excitement that we could form a viable national organization" (Seymour and Smith 1986, 13).

The first symposium was held at the University of California–San Francisco Medical Center on January 31 and February 1, 1970. More than 300 staff and volunteers from the country's sixty-two existing free clinics attended the workshop. During the conference, it became apparent that the clinics were facing similar problems: a lack of sustained funding, inadequate staffing, and difficulties with local authorities and the medical establishment. There was enthusiastic sharing of ideas, sometimes heated exchanges, and an underlying excitement about the emergence of free clinics. The newly formed Executive Committee presented the following draft of a mission statement (Smith, Bentel, and Schwartz 1971, vii–viii):

National Free Clinic Council Statement of Purpose (1971)

All institutions of our society are being confronted by a growing crisis of performance, with bureaucratic process replacing necessary responses to individual and community needs and with organizational control supplanting quality of service. This crisis is highly visible within the health care community in the United States.

The Executive Committee of the National Free Clinic Council believes that quality health care is a right of every individual, not a privilege dependent upon socioeconomic status, social ethic, or geographical location. We further believe that quality alternatives to existing methods of health care must be developed and implemented in order to make available both facilities and personnel for those individuals who are defined or who define themselves as medically indigent.

We believe that health care transcends clinical medicine. Health for an individual depends on fulfillment of basic human needs, both physical and mental.

Health services, therefore, should be provided for all people within a context of total health—individual, community, and social health. Total health care implies adequate personnel and facilities, full access to services, and a major new emphasis on preventive medicine via public education, all of which should involve the community being served in both planning and implementation of its local health care system.

Within the past four years a unique concept of community-based health care has evolved into an explicit attempt to resolve some important aspects of the crisis of performance in health care. . . . The free clinic "movement" has become part of the massive change now occurring within the health care community. The National Free Clinic Council has the following operational objectives:

1. To provide a focal point for the sociomedical momentum of the free clinic "movement."
2. To develop and maintain a system of information dissemination concerning all aspects of free clinic operation.
3. To gain access to health care funding which is available at the national level and to distribute such monies equally to member free clinics.
4. To sponsor and administer an annual National Free Clinic Council Symposium.
5. To provide consultation services both for improvement of quality of services being rendered in established free clinics and for establishment and organization of new free clinics.

The National Free Clinic Council will not assume any administrative control of individual free clinics, the autonomy of each facility must be preserved in order to define, confront, and effectively deal with each community's needs.

The future goal of the National Free Clinic Council is to overcome the crisis orientation of most of the currently operational free clinics. The critical unfulfilled needs in drug abuse, venereal disease, birth control and abortion, malnutrition, and dental health are now requiring full attention of most free clinics. The attainment of national legitimization for free clinics will aid in eliminating some of the desperate quality pervading the operation of such facilities at the present time and permit the necessary expansion into all primary health care services.

Executive Committee
National Free Clinic Council
David E. Smith, M.D., President
James N. Oss, Executive Director
Thomas Payte, M.D.
Alan Reed, M.D.
Joseph Brenner, M.D.
Leon Fay
Gerald DeAngelis, Ph.D.
Edmund Zerkin
Arnie Leff, M.D.
Lawrence Halpern, Ph.D.
David Bearman, M.D.
Joy Balzer

One of the hotly debated issues at the symposium was the desirability of having a national association. Many thought that a national association would be an effective means for collecting and disseminating information on problems being experienced by young people, especially drug problems, and on humane ways of providing treatment. Others were most enthused about having a communication channel for free clinics. Still others were most excited about the potential of a national association for obtaining funding from government and private sources to help secure the financial feasibility of clinics. Many of the clinics represented at the symposium indicated that they were bordering on financial collapse (Seymour and Smith 1986).

But many in the audience were opposed to a national association. The lack of bureaucratic organization was an important source of pride for many free clinics, and a national association—even of free clinics themselves—seemed antithetical to this value. There was also opposition expressed to the idea of trying to obtain government funding. This was a time when social activism and countercultural ideas were at a high pitch, and there was widespread and intense hostility toward the Nixon Administration and toward government agencies such as the FBI and the CIA. It had come to light that the FBI was infiltrating groups, such as the peace movement and the civil rights movement, that opposed administration policies. Fear was expressed that government funding would be a conduit in which the government could infiltrate free clinics and destroy them from the inside.

A third source of opposition was the perception held by some that David Smith and the Haight-Ashbury Free Clinic were overly involved in the formation of the association. Several of the clinics had established completely decentralized decision-making structures in an attempt to avoid a top-heavy (that is, top-down) administration. Some perceived that the Haight-Ashbury Clinic had assumed too much leadership in the effort to create a national association, and they objected to the fact that the first executive committee was essentially self-appointed (Seymour and Smith 1986).

These differences overlapped with what emerged as a major philosophical division among the clinics. Some envisioned the core commitment to be the provision of humane and nonjudgmental quality medical care for anyone in need (Richard Seymour and David Smith refer to clinics adopting this position as "counterculture, service-oriented clinics"), while others viewed the essence of free clinics as being the starting point for revolutionary changes in the health care delivery system (called by Seymour and Smith "radical political clinics"). Though this is an oversimplification, the first group prioritized medical objectives, while the second group emphasized political objectives.

Conversation about what the free clinic movement ought to be continued for the next year and came to a head at the Second National Free Clinic Council Symposium, held at the Shoreham Hotel in Washington, DC, in January 1972. This second symposium ultimately led to the demise of a national association.

THE FALL OF THE NATIONAL FREE CLINIC COUNCIL

Strong feelings dominated the gathering from the time it was planned and scheduled. Many things contributed to the highly charged atmosphere. . . . Pfizer Pharmaceuticals allocated $20,000 for NFCC to cover speakers' honoraria and travel, hotel expenses, publicity, operational expenses, etc. While this money was a godsend to the NFCC organization, some of the clinic representatives considered pharmaceutical companies even more of a devil than the federal government. To them, the Pfizer money was doubly tainted. They wanted no part if it, yet they objected when the NFCC tightened its regulations on whose travel and expenses would be paid. The choice of the Shoreham Hotel, labeled by some as "one of D.C.'s more conservative places," rankled, as did the organizers' "obvious elitism" in not furnishing a list of places in Washington where attendees could crash for free. (Seymour and Smith 1986, 140)

The issue of government funding resurfaced at this second meeting as word spread that David Smith had been negotiating with the federal government for a $1 million grant to the NFCC. During the year between the first and second symposia, the Department of Health, Education, and Welfare and some members of Congress had expressed strong support for the concept of free health clinics and had communicated a willingness to offer sizable funding. David Smith and the NFCC Executive Council arranged to meet with representatives from the National Institutes of Mental Health while they were in town for the Free Clinic Symposium.

Announcement of this meeting provoked anger among those opposed to government funding and further suspicion of the Haight-Ashbury Free Clinic, which had been awarded an eight-year, $320,000 drug treatment grant from NIMH (National Institute of Mental Health) in the previous year. The conference itself was emblematic of the times: harsh rhetoric among individuals whose shared dedication to free clinics was matched by political and philosophical differences.

Ultimately, it was representatives of the Black Caucus, many of whom represented neighborhood clinics, who inspired some resolution. On the last day of the symposium, a clear difference had settled in between those seeing free clinics mostly in medical terms and those seeing the clinics primarily in terms of their political potential. One of the representatives of the Black Caucus addressed the group this way:

Cut the bullshit. . . . You white guys can play your politics, and, if you lose, and your clinic closes, you can go shave your beards and cut your hair and go get good medical care anywhere. We can't, and we need those clinics. (quoted in Seymour and Smith 1986, 142)

While some clinics continued to oppose government funding, the minority clinics (including those run by the Black Panthers) favored application for federal money and joined forces with David Smith and the NFCC Executive Committee. This alliance prevailed, gave direction to the organization, and clearly established service to underserved populations as the primary thrust of free clinics. At the conclusion of the meeting, David Smith resigned as president of the NFCC but became a member of the newly constituted Executive Committee.

Despite this resolution and its framework for change in the ensuing years, the seeds for the ultimate demise of the national association were planted at the symposium. On the morning after the symposium ended, the new committee met with Dr. John Kramer of the President's Special Action Office for Drug Abuse Prevention. At this meeting, it was made clear that the federal government was willing to provide a million-dollar grant to support free clinics and that it wished to do so as soon as possible.

Following this meeting and an exchange of messages between the NFCC and NIMH, the NFCC Ad Hoc Executive Committee met on February 25 to determine whether or not to accept the grant. Representatives of the more politically focused clinics were still opposed and had vehemently expressed their opposition in letters to the NFCC Executive Committee, David Smith, and NIMH. Nevertheless, after considerable debate, the executive committee voted fifteen to one to accept the grant with the proviso that four conditions be acceptable. The provisions largely were designed to ensure that the federal government would not be able to control free clinics. The executive committee then wrote to each of the existing free clinics to report acceptance of the grant, to acknowledge shortcomings in the representativeness of the previous committee, and to initiate a new, more representative selection method. David Smith, who made it clear that he had accepted no salary from either the Haight-Ashbury Free Clinic or the NFCC, distanced himself from policy making to try to further calm the atmosphere (Seymour and Smith 1986).

One final storm erupted as details of the grant were determined. The federal government did not want to deal with each clinic individually but insisted upon dealing with an existing nonprofit corporation with a history of fiscal responsibility. The only available entity (NFCC was not incorporated at this time) that met all of the government requirements was Youth Projects, Inc., a program run by the Haight-Ashbury Free Clinic. The government was willing to provide the funds only if Youth Projects accepted responsibility for it. The executive committee concluded that meeting this requirement was necessary in order to receive the funding, but doing so created a new firestorm of hostility about the dominant role of the Haight-Ashbury Clinic.

As it turned out, Youth Projects was never entirely comfortable with the arrangement and responsibilities, and David Smith continued to urge the NFCC to incorporate and take over responsibility for the grant. In 1976, partly due to the efforts of Sarah Dowdy, the new leader of Youth Projects, the NFCC incorporated. Ironically, shortly thereafter, the new NFCC Executive Committee decided to accept no further federal funds. With no funds to support activities, and with individual free clinics focused on their own efforts to achieve financial stability, the National Free Clinic Council ceased to function (Seymour and Smith 1986).

> Definitely, at the beginning, there was support for a national free clinic movement. When the Washington Conference for free clinics came together, NIMH decided it wanted to fund and encourage free clinics to develop the National Free Clinic Council. They wanted to provide two things: a means for supporting a national organization around free clinics and providing training funding for free clinic personnel, mainly around drug treatment, and providing a communication system with a national newsletter and national files of information on the free clinics.
>
> One of the basic problems was that the government insisted that the funding go through an organization that they could deal with directly instead of dealing with each free clinic individually. It had to be an agency with a track record and responsibility. They looked at Youth Projects, Inc., which was part of the Haight-Ashbury Clinics, so we ended up being the fiscal body that oversaw the grant. This had its good points and its bad points. Think about the wide range of white radical free clinics that existed at this time, putting social pressure on the establishment, women's clinics, and minority clinics. Even though these clinics had a radical agenda as well, the overriding political agenda was the desire to provide medical care for African American communities across the country, and as a consequence, they were the most organized and most interested in seeing a national organization.
>
> With such a wide range of groups, there were, of course, people who resented whomever was holding the purse strings. There was always a fair amount of looking at David and the National Free Clinic Council as a hierarchy of being some sort of tyrannical outfit, while at the same time, David and I were just running around saying, "Hey, we are just a free clinic like everybody else. We just happened to be standing there when they threw the ball." The council ran along until 1976, and then we made a major effort along with representatives from various clinics to help the NFCC to incorporate, so that they would be freestanding. There was much discussion.
>
> Finally, the NFCC was incorporated, and one of the first things that the new corporation did was tell the federal government that they did not want any more funding. The first movement as a national movement, in my opinion, lost something by doing that. (Richard Seymour, Director of Training and Education, Haight-Ashbury Free Clinics, San Francisco, California)

YEARS OF ISOLATION

The negative feelings engendered by the national symposia and the collapse of the National Free Clinic Council touched most or all of the individuals involved. When the NFCC ceased operating, the last thing that most wanted was any new form of collective organization. While some contacts made at the symposia continued, and while David Smith continued to share the Haight-Ashbury Free Clinic's experiences in writing and consultation, most free clinics simply went their own way.

To illustrate this isolation, in 1982, I conducted research that required me to identify all of the free health clinics in the southeastern section of the country and all of the clinics that had existed but had closed in the previous five years. There were no central registries, and trying to identify existing and closed clinics was an arduous task. I searched telephone directories, made telephone calls to state departments of health and to local public health departments and to various other health agencies. When I contacted a free clinic directly, I asked for information about other free clinics in the same city, in the same state, and in the region. No one had extensive knowledge of the existence of other free clinics. Some clinics that had been around since the early days—for example, the Fan Free Clinic in Richmond, Virginia, and the Corner Drug Store in Gainesville, Florida—were known by name by several individuals. But no one had any idea how many free clinics existed in their home state, and free clinics in Atlanta—the city with the most free clinics in the region at that time—were unaware of other free clinics in the same city.

An outgrowth of the contacts made in this research project was a regional free health clinic symposium held in Atlanta in 1983. Roanoke's Bradley Free Clinic organized and sponsored the conference, and almost all of the southeastern free clinics sent representatives. The conference focused strongly on sharing knowledge, experiences, and expertise in the day-to-day management of a free clinic and de-emphasized discussion of free health clinics as a revolutionary political movement. There was generally a very positive spirit that prevailed at the conference. Most attendees felt that they acquired some valuable information and made some good contacts, although differences in clinic philosophy (for example, the necessity of eligibility requirements) and clinic structure (for example, the size of the pharmacy) were apparent.

However, there was little interest in creating a formal, regional association or in any kind of organizational structure. There was interest in getting together again for another conference as long as one or more of the most established clinics would take the lead but not for anything more than that. The reluctance was based on two factors. First, lingering stories about the experience of the National Free Clinic Council (although almost no one at the regional meeting had personally been involved with the NFCC or had attended any of its symposia), had many feeling very shy about trying to re-create any formal structure. Second, many of the second-generation free clinics were just getting started in the early 1980s. Travel budgets were almost nonexistent, and clinics were very much focused on day-to-day operations.

I think some of this reluctance was driven by the free clinics that came into being in the late 1960s and early 1970s. When this clinic was started in 1982, it was
the first free clinic in West Virginia. At that point, you are fighting so much to
keep your head above water. It is not like you have a huge amount of funds
coming in like a federally qualified health center. You are really fighting to serve
the patients and to expand your hours so that you are more reliable and are
viewed by the patients as a place to go for services. The focus of the clinic is
very much internal rather than external. (Patricia Holmes White, Executive Director of West Virginia Health Right, Charleston, West Virginia)

In most areas of the country there was not any effort to meet together or
to establish any kind of information network. From the time of the dissolu-
tion of the NFCC in 1976 until the formation of a statewide association of free
clinics in Virginia during 1991 and 1992, there were no state, regional, or national associations of free health clinics.

ORGANIZING AT THE STATE AND REGIONAL LEVELS

The Virginia Association of Free Clinics (VAFC)

While California's free clinics have participated for several years in a consortium with community health clinics, Virginia was the first state to develop
an association strictly for free clinics. The fact that this happened in Virginia
may be unsurprising. Virginia was home to two long-standing, well-
established free clinics (in Richmond and Roanoke). The Fan Free Clinic in
Richmond was a large free clinic that offered a wide range of services, had
strong community support, and had a solid volunteer base. It was one of the
few 1960s-generation free clinics that had survived and thrived. The Bradley
Free Clinic in Roanoke had been started in 1974 and had secured a strong
base in its home community. Estelle Nichols Avner, executive director of the
Bradley Free Clinic, had for several years tirelessly and without compensation travelled to communities around the state (and region) assisting interested groups in creating a free clinic. Avner and the Bradley Free Clinic
Board of Directors had sponsored regional meetings, established the National Free Clinic Foundation, and had assembled and disseminated a *National Directory of Free Clinics*. Virginia had one other extremely important
thing going for it: a corporation or foundation that was willing to make ongoing significant financial contributions to help develop and sustain free
clinics. Trigon (which had been Blue Cross-Blue Shield of Virginia and is
now Anthem) committed to contributing financially to free clinics throughout Virginia. In the early 1990s, there were just eight free clinics in Virginia,
while today there are forty-seven.

But formation of a statewide association was not an easy process. Even
among the relatively small number of free clinics that existed in Virginia in

the early 1990s, there were very different visions about what a state association should be and how it should be structured. Efforts to form a statewide association began in 1991 but did not lead to incorporation until 1993. Mark Cruise, executive director of the VAFC, recounts that

> the process of starting the Virginia Association actually was quite contentious. It was not a smooth process at all. It took a very long time and a lot of work to build a consensus as to what the purpose of the association would be and how it would operate and be structured and be governed.

The support of Trigon was very important to this process as it helped to fund statewide meetings as well as providing support to individual clinics.

When incorporated, representatives from existing clinics elected a nine-person board of directors to oversee the association. Everything was done on a strictly volunteer basis—initially, there were no paid staff members. The volunteers produced a newsletter and organized an annual meeting. A part-time person was hired in 1996, but the need for a full-time director quickly became apparent. Mark Cruise, who had experience working with CHIP (the Child Health Investment Partnership), a public-private agency designed to increase access to services for Medicaid children and families, and as executive director of the New River Valley (Christiansburg, Virginia) Free Health Clinic, was hired as the full-time director and began work in 1997. The formal mission statement and objectives of the VAFC and its primary activities are provided in the accompanying boxes. Membership in the VAFC is open to "independent, private, nonprofit, community-based organizations that operate a volunteer-driven free clinic or 'clinic without walls' that primarily serves low-income, uninsured Virginians" (see www.vafreeclinics.org/ab-mem-p.html).

In its short history, the VAFC has assembled an impressive list of accomplishments. It collects data from clinics on an annual basis. Every clinic has been assisted in having access to e-mail. Liability plans for executive directors and for health care professional groups have been purchased. In fiscal year 1999, for the first time, through efforts by the VAFC, the state appropriated funds ($600,000) for free clinics. By fiscal year 2002, the size of this appropriation passed the million-dollar mark ($1.08 million). State funding has been earmarked for pharmacy services—the biggest financial need of the clinics. Free clinics have leveraged this money into dramatically larger services: for every dollar spent on a free clinic pharmacy, seven dollars of prescription medicines is provided to the low-income, uninsured population. VAFC efforts now make it possible for free clinics to purchase medical and dental supplies off the state contract (which provides a sizable discount and enables free clinic funds to reach further). The list of professionals who can get a tax credit for contributions to free clinics has been expanded.

Virginia Association of Free Clinics: Mission Statement, Objectives, and Services

Mission Statement:
The Virginia Association of Free Clinics is a membership organization whose mission is to strengthen and support free clinics and advocate for the populations they serve.

Objectives:
1. To increase networking among member clinics.
2. To keep member clinics updated on various state and national public policy Issues and legislation affecting health care.
3. To collect and disseminate aggregate data and information for the purpose of the development of public policy and legislation that affects the population we serve, thereby giving a stronger voice to those we serve.
4. To provide cost-saving opportunities to member clinics through group purchasing opportunities and the leveraging of in-kind gifts.
5. To encourage and contribute to the development of regional and national free clinic associations.
6. To encourage high standards of operation for member clinics, professionalism for their staff members, and excellence in their governing bodies.
7. To provide educational opportunities for member clinic staff and board members.
8. To develop and encourage the use of communications vehicles such as a newsletter, e-mail connections, and other means.
9. To develop and maintain relationships with other public, private, and professional health-related organizations.
10. To provide technical assistance to member clinics and those interested in starting new clinics.

Services:
The VAFC provides the following services:
1. An annual conference of Virginia's free clinics (the meeting rotates around the state, and attendees are able to visit nearby free clinics)
2. Collection and compilation of data on Virginia's free clinics
3. Publication of the Resource Manual for Virginia's Free Clinics
4. Monitoring and analysis of health policy and regulations
5. Legislative advocacy on behalf of free clinics
6. Funding (the VAFC serves as the fiscal agent for state and other funds earmarked for free clinics)
7. Technical assistance and consultation for member clinics and communities interested in starting a free clinic (the VAFC assists communities that are starting a free clinic)
8. An annual retreat for free clinic executive directors
9. Representation for free clinics on the Virginia Quality Healthcare Network, Virginia Coalition on Children's Health, Virginians for Improving Access to Dental Care, Virginians for a Healthy Future, and the Coalition of Virginia Nonprofits
10. An annual free clinic clinical coordinators workday
11. Regular membership update on matters of interest to free clinics
12. Peer support and networking
13. Public relations and marketing

Through its documentation of need, the VAFC has convinced Trigon (Anthem) to continue its annual support of free clinics. In the early 1990s, Trigon annually contributed $25,000 to each Virginia free clinic. As the number of free clinics grew rapidly, Trigon decided to ratchet the annual per clinic contribution down to $20,000, then $15,000, then $10,000, and then to discontinue it altogether. Instead, Trigon has now decided to maintain the $10,000-per-year contribution to each clinic and to support other clinic activities. Its annual contribution exceeds $500,000.

The North Carolina Association of Free Clinics (NCAFC)

In 1998, North Carolina became the second state to have an incorporated statewide free clinic association. Like Virginia, North Carolina was represented in the first generation of free clinics (in Chapel Hill and Durham), had several very well established free clinics located throughout the state, had benefited from having some free clinic directors who assisted other communities in creating their own free clinic, and had significant support from large private foundations (for example, the Kate B. Reynolds Charitable Trust and the Duke Endowment). North Carolina's location bordering Virginia also facilitated cooperation and exchange between the states.

Since 2000, the NCAFC has been led by John Mills. As with Mark Cruise in Virginia, Mills had extensive experience with free clinics in that he had served as Pharmacy Director at Crisis Control Ministry Clinic (CCMC) in Winston-Salem, North Carolina. The CCMC is one of a small number of free clinics nationally (though there are several in North Carolina) that focus on the provision of free medications to those who cannot afford them and who do not have insurance that will pay for them. It is a largely volunteer-driven clinic that does not accept government funds. In the year 2000, when John became director of the NCAFC, the CCMC dispensed more than 38,000 prescriptions—a value of $1.4 million in wholesale drugs—on a budget of $350,000. John's experiences in working with the community, other free clinics, professional associations, higher education institutions, and the state legislature offered a valuable base for the statewide association.

The NCAFC carefully drafted a mission statement, a vision statement, an explication of its core values, and its specific objectives (see the accompanying insert).

By 2004, there were fifty-seven free health clinics in North Carolina; forty-nine provide comprehensive primary care and some specialty care (more than twenty provide emergency dental care), and eight provide strictly pharmacy assistance. In the year 2002 alone, North Carolina's free clinics provided more than $60 million of free health care services to more than 125,000 patients. More than 6,000 health care professionals and other community citizens volunteered their time to the free clinics, and more than $9 million was raised from the private sector (see www.ncfreeclinics.org).

The North Carolina Association of Free Clinics: Mission, Vision, and Core Values

Mission Statement:
To serve as an advocate for member free clinics and the populations they serve.

Vision:
A collaborative network to improve access to health care for the uninsured and underinsured people of North Carolina.

Core Values:
- We believe that inability to pay should not prevent people from receiving health care.
- We believe that all health care is "local" and that community-based planning, governance, and collaboration are critical.
- We believe that good stewardship of resources means obtaining donated equipment, supplies, and services whenever possible.
- We believe that all persons deserve to be treated with dignity and respect.

Source: www.ncfreeclinics.org/about_us.htm

On January 14, 2004, the NCAFC announced a $10 million partnership with the Blue Cross and Blue Shield of North Carolina Foundation to strengthen and expand services to the state's uninsured and underinsured. The grant, which will be distributed over five years, provides an annual allocation of $15,000 to each existing free clinic; a pool of funds to support expansion of existing services; money to purchase the flu vaccine; awards for excellence in the areas of innovation, use of technology, and the elimination of racial and ethnic health disparities; and planning grants, infrastructure grants, and start-up grants for new free clinics. This is, by far, the single biggest grant received by free clinics and one that signifies a belief by Blue Cross and Blue Shield of North Carolina that free clinics are one of the answers to providing health care coverage for the uninsured and underinsured (North Carolina Association of Free Clinics).

Free Clinics of the Great Lakes Region

In December 1996, free health clinic representatives from Illinois, Indiana, Iowa, Michigan, and Ohio organized the first-of-its-kind regional network of free health clinics—the Free Clinics of the Great Lakes Region (FCGLR). The proposed network received a grant of $6,900 from the W. K. Kellogg Foundation to fund a conference for all of the free clinics in the region and to enable them to create a formal association. The conference occurred in April 1997 and focused on ways that the clinics, despite their differences in structure and targeted services, could work together for their mutual benefit and to enhance their ability to provide health care for the uninsured. Representatives from more than twenty-five clinics attended the conference.

Subsequent conferences were held in 1998 (with more than forty clinics represented) and in 1999 (with more than fifty clinics represented). A 1999 survey, "Assessing the Impact of the Free Clinics of the Great Lakes Region," conducted by the Robert Wood Johnson Foundation–funded Volunteers in Health Care, was instrumental in identifying existing free clinics and supporting their organization. An additional grant by the W. K. Kellogg Foundation of $38,000 further facilitated development of the regional association.

The primary leader of this regional effort has been Jane Zwiers, a registered nurse, who has been and is the executive director of the First Presbyterian Church Health Clinic in Kalamazoo, Michigan. As director of that clinic, Zwiers has had extensive work with identifying the health care needs of the uninsured, working with other community organizations, marshaling a large professional and lay volunteer pool (today, numbering more than 350), and overseeing the needs of the clinic. She saw the benefits of a regional network and became the driving force in its inception.

> We started a regional effort to support each other, to nurture each other, to help each other, and to learn from each other, not to have to reinvent the wheel. It is a genuine grassroots relationship. We realized how much we had in common. We shared materials, nobody charged for anything, and there was no competition. We grew and grew and grew. Now, each state also has its own coordinator. We do strategic planning, mentoring, maintain a Web site and Listserv, assist in partnering with other agencies in the community, and promote the visibility of clinics. The Kellogg Foundation was extremely helpful in the early years— they were a wonderfully supportive liaison. Then, Volunteers in Health Care also helped the regional to strengthen the association. VIHC now is aiding our medication access. In November 2000, we created Volume Rx, a bulk buying consortium, that enables clinics to purchase supplies at much lower cost. For example, clinics were paying $28 per albuterol inhaler—now it is $4.67. We are now doing much more systematic data collection trying to really track the uninsured for their clinical needs. (Jane Zwiers, Executive Director, First Presbyterian Church Health Clinic, Kalamazoo, Michigan)

Today, there are more than 200 clinics in the FCGLR (which includes the original five states plus Minnesota and Wisconsin) (see www.fcglr.net).

INCREASING DEVELOPMENT OF STATE ASSOCIATIONS

During the last few years, several additional statewide free health clinic associations have been created. The Vermont Coalition of Clinics for the Uninsured (VCCU)—a group of nine free primary health clinics and one free dental clinic—was created in 1995. The clinics meet on a quarterly basis, use common software for data collection to enable the most accurate monitoring of health care needs throughout the state, and sponsor a Web site (www.vccu.net). The South Carolina Free Medical Clinic Association (SCFMCA) began in 2001. The SCFMCA is sponsored by the South Carolina Hospital Association but has a separate board of directors. It also has extended significant effort in data collection and has partnered with the Office of Research and Statistics of the South Carolina Budget and Control Board to develop a single free clinic database. The SCFMCA sponsors an annual conference, ongoing continuing education projects, and a Web site. The Ohio Association of Free Clinics was created in 2002 and provides significant statewide networking in addition to the regional networking enabled by the Free Clinics of the Great Lakes Region Association. West Virginia's free clinics have met together formally and informally for several years and created a formal statewide association in 2003. Statewide associations have now been developed in Georgia, Iowa, Illinois, Indiana, Kentucky, Louisiana, Michigan, Minnesota, Missouri, Texas, and Wisconsin. A second regional association, Free Clinics of the Western Region (including clinics in Arizona, California, Idaho, Oregon, Utah, and Washington), has also been developed.

Part of this momentum comes from the success and modeling of the Virginia and North Carolina state associations. Part of the success is also due to the availability of funding to support the development of state free clinic associations from the Robert Wood Johnson Foundation–funded Volunteers in Health Care.

It made a difference when Volunteers in Health Care, an outgrowth of the Robert Wood Johnson ReachOut Project, started putting dollars into support for state associations. It was a way for them to develop a base of knowledge for volunteers to call and to get assistance. When those dollars were put out, it enabled a lot of free clinics to try to formalize a state association. It helped to subsidize opportunities for clinic staffs to get together, whereas before only clinic directors had gotten together. (Patricia Holmes White, Executive Director of West Virginia Health Right, Charleston, West Virginia)

Issues in Developing State and Regional Associations

The development of state and regional free clinic associations has enjoyed widespread support. Although the process by which these associations have developed differs, states and regions around the country have been able to learn from the early experiences in Virginia, North Carolina, and the Great Lakes region.

The concerns that have arisen about these collective organizations generally focus around two themes: the potential sacrifice of independence for individual free clinics and the potential negative consequences of structures of bureaucracy and political authority. Free health clinic staff and volunteers are acutely aware of how hard they have worked to gain acceptance and stability within their own communities. Most believe strongly that their freedom in creating and developing the clinic was essential in their success. They value their independence and, for the most part, have reservations about any kind of organizational setup that would impose standards or regulations from agents outside the community. Thus, those involved in developing state associations have found it necessary to work with this independent spirit of individual clinics and to devise ways to accrue the benefits of state (or regional) association without stepping over this boundary.

Jim Beckner, executive director of the Fan Free Clinic in Richmond, Virginia, and an important advocate for the formation of free clinic collective associations, expresses this key idea:

> We are all very different and yet we also have things on which we are all the same. We are all community-based. With that comes a fierce independence and accountability to self and community. It is easy to take the view that we are not accountable to the entire state or to other communities—that we have had to fight and scrap and scrounge for this clinic and prove ourself as an organization from the ground up. That attracts fiercely independent, pig-headed directors like myself. . . . But these are the very things that make our individual clinics successful in the communities where we are located. In Virginia, we spent a number of years just getting to know one another, networking, and exchanging information. We had to learn to trust one another before the state association could really get moving. In the early days there was discussion about taking a position on national health care, and I asked that no one bring that up in a public forum because it could be divisive. We avoided that like the plague. Now, the association has proved its worth so that the members now see value in what we can accomplish together.

At some point, each collective association has addressed the issue of having statewide standards or regulations. Some free clinics see advantages to this: enhanced quality control, a stimulus for clinic improvements, increased clinic credibility, and so forth. Others have opposed the implementation of standards. One difficulty pointed out is that clinics vary so much in their structure, their access to community resources, and their patient focus.

> I'm not sure how we can develop standards that apply to every clinic because free clinics spring out of community need, and they all come about with a different group of people and with a different sense of resources. Not every clinic has access to a health care system like I do. Some have a lot more, but many have less. (Jeri White, Executive Director, The Community Clinic of High Point, High Point, North Carolina, and a key advocate for collective association)

The issue of statewide standards also has arisen with respect to the issue of use of common data collection methods by all of the clinics. This issue has been considered in many of the associations, and on each of these occasions, some have strongly supported standardized data collection, while others have strongly opposed it. There is a fairly wide sense that free clinics could make a more powerful statement about the health care needs of the uninsured and working poor and about the contributions of free health clinics if there was more systematic data collection. Jane Zwiers, among others, feels that the credibility of the free clinic movement has suffered due to lack of good data. But, at this point, associations have made conflicting decisions—some associations have chosen not to establish a common database, while others have opted to do so.

South Carolina is a state that is developing a single database. The decision was made to collect data that would be helpful in understanding state health care needs *and* would be helpful to individual clinics. The database was created with contributions from individual clinics, and pilot tested, modified, and implemented in all of the clinics that belong to the state association. Clinics report on a quarterly basis to the Office of Research and Statistics of the South Carolina Budget and Control Board, whose statisticians analyze the data and report results to the clinics.

Overlapping with the concern about loss of independence is a concern about the creation of bureaucracy that will create excessive time demands on clinics and possibly lead to a diminution of the camaraderie that typically exists among free clinic staff and volunteers. The question raised is not whether something like a common database is helpful but whether or not it justifies the amount of time required to participate. Barb Tylenda, executive director of the Health Care Network, Inc., in Racine, Wisconsin, has represented Wisconsin in the Free Clinics of the Great Lakes Region and supports the move toward a re-creation of a national association. At the same time, she expresses a concern shared by many:

> The support provided by the regional association is wonderful. It is nice to have someone who speaks your language and with whom you can talk. Clinics are all at different stages, but no matter what stage one is at, there is always some little tip that someone can offer that is helpful. Even the way that someone phrases things might make a light bulb go on. You learn what resources are out there. The association helps more people learn about free clinics, and the more that is known, the more likely they are to contribute funds. But the potential disadvantage of associations is that they can turn into a power struggle—that we have individuals who want more to be president as opposed to right now where people just want to do the right thing. We could start arguing about things that in the whole scope of things really aren't that important, but they get elevated to a new level because of the organization.

Perceived Benefits of Collective Association

Despite these concerns, more and more states are moving to establish a collective association. What are the primary benefits that members identify?

Networking

The most commonly identified benefit of belonging to a state or regional free clinic association is the opportunity to network with other clinics. Clinic staff and volunteers speak glowingly of the interaction with others who understand free clinics from the inside; the resources that are freely shared; the chance to question, vent, and commiserate; and the feelings of belonging to a group with a common focus.

> Our goal in the North Carolina Free Clinic Association is first and foremost to be a network, to be a united voice. Second, we want to provide education. We are unique in medicine. There is nothing else out there like what we do. While we practice medicine, we do it differently. Sometimes, I remind my physicians that you have to go back and do it like you used to. We're there to help the free clinics pull it together. We provide education for directors and staff; two retreats for directors each year plus an annual meeting. These are huge events with speakers and topics that are relevant to the free clinic world like accessing medication assistance programs, eligibility, and marketing. (Sandy Motley, Executive Director, Davidson Medical Ministries Clinic, Inc., Lexington, North Carolina)

> The Virginia Association has been fantastic for all of us. The state network is so wonderful. The annual executive directors' retreat is a lifesaver. We get many good ideas from the annual conference. Plus, now, there is on-line help. If we want to develop a new policy, we simply get on-line and ask for help. The sense of isolation that has traditionally existed in free clinics has been removed. (Becky Weybright, Executive Director, Charlottesville Free Clinic, Charlottesville, Virginia)

> A few years ago, the free clinics in New England got together for a meeting. It became clear that however well one is doing, there is always something more that can be learned if you listen to what other people are doing. So many states are well organized with incredible state associations. (Karen Gottlieb, Americares Free Clinics, New Canaan, Connecticut)

> The Great Lakes Association has been wonderful. We are in constant contact with them. There is one state meeting each year and one regional conference. The networking is very helpful. If we have a problem, we contact others and ask about how they are handling it. It may be about volunteers or fund-raising or collective buying. There isn't any downside for us. (Cam Buenzli, Healthnet of Janesville, Inc., Janesville, Wisconsin)

I believe wholeheartedly that coming together will help you to achieve some things. One of the key benefits is the support and knowledge you get from neighboring clinics. North Carolina is sufficiently organized now that we have conferences. I have yet to go to a meeting where I haven't learned something. There is a lot of exchange and a lot of support, because usually when you work in a free clinic situation, you are the only one of your kind at a meeting. And very few people outside free clinics really understand the day-to-day decisions that must be made in a free clinic. (Jeri White, Executive Director, The Community Clinic of High Point, High Point, North Carolina)

Free clinics located in states without a free clinic association rarely have the same type of supportive network. Many free clinics in California belong to local community clinic associations that comprise both free and sliding-scale clinics. These associations provide helpful interaction and support. However, clinics operated on a sliding-scale fee basis and free clinics have many different issues as well, and the kind of collective identification that occurs in all–free clinic associations often is absent.

Free clinics in Washington, DC, are in a similar situation. There is a Non-Profit Clinic Consortium, a group of about ten clinics that serve low-income patient groups. The group meets about once per month and works together to try to effect change in the city. But not all of the clinics are free clinics; each is unique in some ways and represents a somewhat different approach, and it is not always easy to secure agreement on policy positions (for example, endorsement or opposition to a city program or legislative bill).

Fund-Raising

The success of the Virginia Association of Free Clinics in obtaining an annual allocation for free clinics from the state government and in securing annual donations from Anthem and the success of the North Carolina Association of Free Clinics in partnering with Blue Cross and Blue Shield of North Carolina are obvious illustrations of the value of collective association for fund-raising. The funds received have been very helpful to all clinics within the state and indispensable for some.

I love the fact that in the state of Virginia we have a director of the state association and that we have made such inroads that we were able to get legislators this past year to fund free clinic pharmacies for $1.3 million. Free clinic folks worked with legislators in their own community and made presentations to the general assembly. Each was so well accepted in their own community that the legislators acknowledged that the clinics really are doing something important to help the quality of life of their patients. (Estelle Nichols Avner, Executive Director, Bradley Free Clinic, Roanoke, Virginia)

The state association has played a tremendous role in our success. We have reaped many benefits from the money given by the state. The state director has really made it happen. We now look very professional. There has also been significant technical assistance. The money that was provided by the Virginia Health Care Foundation for the directors to obtain some kind of advanced health care management education showed a lot of foresight and enabled directors to take their clinics to a much higher level. (Linda Cornelius, Executive Director, Augusta Regional Free Clinic, Fishersville, Virginia)

The Virginia Association of Free Clinics has provided wonderful support, guidance, and a wealth of knowledge. . . . We could not survive without the financial help that they have obtained and provided. (Marilynn Bridges, Executive Director, and Karon Jones, Clinical Services Director, Free Clinic of Franklin County, Rocky Mount, Virginia)

Group Purchasing

Some of the associations have emphasized the development of group purchasing programs for member clinics. The underlying idea is straightforward. Many medical supplies are sold at a per unit cost, and the larger the number purchased, the smaller the per unit price. Typically, individual free clinics only require a small number of needed supplies, and thus they pay a high per unit price. Statewide or regional associations can serve as a conduit for purchasing supplies for the collectivity of free clinics within their area. This enables a larger volume to be purchased, meaning a smaller per unit cost, and substantial savings to individual clinics. It is another way that free clinics can stretch the available dollars to provide the maximum amount of services.

The Volume Rx program of the Free Clinics of the Great Lakes Region association illustrates this type of bulk purchasing program. Member clinics can submit orders for supplies through a simple link on the association Web site; the Kalamazoo (Michigan) Free Clinic serves as the bulk ordering agent; and individual clinics pay less than the standard retail amount for needed supplies.

Public Awareness

Many free clinic staff and volunteers believe that there is much more to do in bringing attention to the contributions of free clinics. Individual clinic staff often devote much time to speaking at events sponsored by civic groups, churches and other religious organizations, local government bodies, and so forth. Information about free clinics is also spread through a myriad of private conversations. However, many believe that collective organizations have the potential to increase significantly the public awareness of clinics. And, collective associations routinely accept this as a responsibility.

Data Collection

If the summary statistics for the contributions of individual free clinics are impressive, the aggregate statistics for free clinics within a state or region can be even more powerful. Routinely, collective associations have taken strides to improve data collection within free clinics and, sometimes, to standardize data collection procedures and reporting, so that valid and reliable aggregate data can be calculated. These data can be especially impressive to potential public and private funding agencies as they document not only the need for services and the contributions of free clinics but also systematic organization within clinics.

Legislative Impact

Over the last decade or two, some free clinic individuals have been asked to testify in state legislatures and even congressional committees. They have brought the potential of free health clinics to a significantly wider audience and they have had some legislative impact. Collective associations likely offer greater potential for two reasons. First, association staff members may have as designated job responsibilities getting to know legislators, having periodic interaction with them, monitoring legislative needs of free clinics, and examining proposed legislation for seen or unforeseen consequences for free clinics. Given the extraordinary demands in running a free clinic, it is very difficult or impossible for any executive director to devote the same attention and activities to working with the legislature. Second, association officers can speak as a representative of a collection of free clinics located in legislative districts around a state or region and can have a stronger voice because of the larger number of people represented and the number of legislators who have reason to be especially attentive to requests. Typically, there is more power in a collective voice than in an individual voice.

> In addition to helping each other, the state association also should have influence on broader policy as an objective. If it doesn't, then the association has missed its mark. I have been involved in a number of initiatives of free clinics coming together. There is always value in learning from each other and in helping each other. It is all good. But, if that is all there is, an association would not sustain itself. And, the reason is that everyone has limited resources and time. It's nice to go talk to people. It's nice to have that kind of learning experience, but when you are stressed and maxed and strapped, the thought of getting together in another part of the state is the thing that will go. It is easy to think that you just don't have time. But, if the state association hits its mark, it will be because we go beyond that, and we see as its purpose addressing issues that impact the lives of people whom we see. The obvious issue is access. We have an opportunity to put a voice out there for the people that we see here in a way that, if we don't do it, it isn't going to get done. So my vision for the state asso-

ciation is that it will be as much issue-oriented as it will be institution-oriented—that when the policymakers at the state level invite people to come to speak to issues of health care, the free clinic association in this state will be one of the organizations at the table. I think the same could be said for associations in other states. (Marty Hiller, Executive Director, Free Clinic of Greater Cleveland, Cleveland, Ohio)

Another important part of the state association is lobbying. John [Mills, the Executive Director of the North Carolina Association of Free Clinics] is a registered lobbyist with the state. We can monitor what is going on in the legislature and monitor things that are relevant to free clinics so that collectively we can be a voice. I certainly don't have time to sit down and read everything that might impact free clinics or might impact the uninsured, but it is nice to know that someone else is going to do that and send me stuff that I need to know. (Sandy Motley, Executive Director, Davidson Medical Ministries, Inc., Lexington, North Carolina)

New Clinic Start-Up

Prior to the advent of collective free clinic associations, it was common for communities considering the creation of a free clinic to do a couple of things. Often, they would review journal and magazine articles and would find that only a small number of relevant pieces were available. Visiting a successful free clinic was very common, and some of the clinics visited in this research have had dozens of visitors from other communities over the years. It has also been common for a few successful clinic directors to travel to communities during the start-up process. Many have contacted Volunteers in Health Care, the Robert Wood Johnson Foundation group based in Rhode Island, or Volunteers in Medicine, the Jack McConnell group based in South Carolina, or Estelle Avner at the Bradley Free Clinic in Roanoke, Virginia, or David Smith and the folks at the Haight-Ashbury Free Clinic in San Francisco. These individuals and groups, and many others, have served in an important consulting capacity. Interestingly, none of them ever did so for profit or remuneration. The commitment has always been to the patients needing services and to the groups willing to come together to create a free clinic to serve them.

The greater resources available in collective associations—in terms of money, information, designated time, and so forth—enable them to take on much of this responsibility. Clinics just starting continue to be in contact with veteran clinics and often do site visits, but state association staff now are key agents in helping to foster the development of new clinics.

Because we were the first state association and because we have a lot of free clinics in Virginia, one of our objectives is to help communities start a free clinic.

It is very important for us to be able to contribute what we know with communities, with other states, and with the nation. That has been an ethic of free clinics in Virginia and around the country. Free clinics as a group are very willing to share. I think Estelle Avner [of the Bradley Free Clinic in Roanoke] contributed to that ethic because that is what she has done—going around the country speaking and producing the clinic directory and not looking at it as a money-making activity. So we as an association have adopted that same ethic. (Mark Cruise, Executive Director, Virginia Association of Free Clinics)

6

The Reemergence
of a National Association

The real challenge of the national association will be to bring people together, to reach consensus, to build bridges, and to create an organization
where people can work together, and maybe agree or disagree about some
things, but keep moving forward.

(Mark Cruise, Interim Director, National Association of Free Clinics)

THE FOUNDING OF THE NATIONAL
ASSOCIATION OF FREE CLINICS (NAFC)

The rapid growth in the number of free clinics nationally and the success of
the emerging state and regional free clinic associations has recently led to the
creation of a new national association. Preliminary conversations about a national association occurred throughout the second half of the 1990s and the
early years of the new century.

Two initiatives went past the conversation point. One was by Jack Mc-
Connell, the physician who, with the financial help of the Robert Wood Johnson Foundation, started the Volunteers in Medicine Clinic in Hilton Head,
South Carolina, in 1994. McConnell himself has been a tireless worker at his
own clinic and of considerable help to other clinics in getting started (Volunteers in Medicine has helped to start more than twenty free clinics around
the country). He has contended that certain issues—most notably, the elimination of legal liability for health care professionals volunteering in free
clinics—could best be resolved at the national level and that a national
association could be instrumental in this effort. He also advocated for the

networking opportunities that could be stimulated by a national association and for an annual conference.

The other initiative occurred primarily among the leadership of the North Carolina and Virginia State Associations of Free Clinics. During the time when the North Carolina Association was just getting off the ground, Glenn Pierce of the ABCCM (Asheville-Buncombe Community Christian Ministry) Clinic in Asheville and Sandy Motley of Davidson Medical Ministries Clinic in Lexington organized a state conference in Lexington. Estelle Avner of the Bradley Free Clinic in Roanoke, Virginia, attended the conference and helped to inspire the group to form a North Carolina state association. The following year, Mark Cruise, executive director of Virginia's association, attended the North Carolina meeting, and, in the following year, Glenn Pierce attended the Virginia meeting. During informal conversations between the two, including Marty Hiller of the Cleveland Free Clinic in the second year, the idea of a national association was discussed. Marty, who had extensive knowledge of free clinic history and had even attended one of the National Free Clinic Council meetings in the early 1970s, shared some of the problems that had plagued the NFCC.

The group recognized that there were multiple "centers of energy" among free clinics: (1) the Jack McConnell group in Hilton Head, (2) the Bradley Free Clinic in Roanoke led by Estelle Avner and Kevin Kelleher, (3) the Free Clinics of the Great Lakes Region led by Jane Zwiers, (4) the Haight-Ashbury Free Clinics led by David Smith, and (5) the Robert Wood Johnson Foundation–funded Volunteers in Health Care based in Rhode Island. However, the various centers were not of one mind with regard to formation of a national association. Not all were convinced that a national association was necessary or even a good idea. The group discussed several key issues about the manner in which a national association could be created: how the initial leaders would be selected, the extent an association would be organization-focused versus politically focused, and the amount of work that the Hilton Head group had already done in trying to create a national association. From the perspective of the advocates for a national association, the absence of universal support was frustrating. Glenn Pierce, especially, felt that the benefits of a national group were compelling and that its creation was overdue. From the perspective of some of the other energy centers, there were important issues that they believed needed to be raised before actual work on a national association commenced. For a time, it did not appear that the initiative to form a national association would move forward.

Then, a new policy developed by the Food and Drug Administration—a policy that did not intentionally have anything to do with free clinics but that would potentially have a significant and devastating impact upon them—re-created talk of a national association. The policy required new bookkeeping and cataloging methods for all drugs received by medical clinics.

For free clinics, which typically obtain drugs from countless sources and often in very small sample amounts donated by individual physicians, the bookkeeping requirement would have been essentially impossible to meet. The hours required to complete the task would have been enormous. John Mills, the pharmacy director of the Crisis Control Ministry Clinic in Winston-Salem, North Carolina, and the executive director of the North Carolina Free Clinic Association, immediately saw the potentially devastating consequences of the requirement. Mills contacted Anthony Young of the law firm Parker, Wetherick, and Marbury in Washington, DC, to do some pro bono work for free clinics relative to the FDA requirement.

INCORPORATION OF THE NAFC

At the same time, conversations occurred among several free clinic individuals about the importance of clinics taking a united stand against the new regulation. Glenn Pierce, Marty Hiller, Pat White (executive director of West Virginia Health Right in Charleston, West Virginia, and a former member of the West Virginia state legislature), Mark Cruise, and John Mills, with some interaction with Sonja Olson in Vermont and Liz Forer in California, formed what they called the National Task Force on Free Clinics to spearhead an effort to work with FDA staff to alter the new regulation or to exempt free clinics from having to meet it. This group sent a survey to free clinics and received a good response. Extensive conversations with FDA representatives subsequently ensued, and the threatening requirement was removed.

This event reinforced for some the benefits of a national association and persuaded some others that collective organization could be an effective agent to monitor proposed federal legislation that would impact free clinics. As it turned out, some other recently developed FDA regulations were also negatively impacting free clinics, so many perceived an immediate need to proceed. Even among the enthusiastic supporters of a national association, however, there were some differences about the most important next steps. Some wanted to move forward quickly—to create a structure for a national association and to begin acquiring a financial base. Others preferred to build the base of supporting free clinics before moving forward. Something of a compromise was worked out. In April 2001, Glenn Pierce drafted bylaws for a national association that included formation of a board that would have two years to define the structure of the association and to devise a system for obtaining input from other free clinic representatives. In October of that year, at the annual meeting of the Virginia Free Clinic Association, the national association became incorporated as a 501(c)(3) nonprofit organization.

The initial board was comprised of seven individuals: Marty Hiller (president), Pat White (vice president), Liz Forer (secretary), Glenn Pierce (treasurer and interim director), Jim Beckner (of the Fan Free Clinic in Richmond, Virginia), Sheri Wood (of the Kansas City, Missouri, Free Health Clinics), and Karen Gottlieb (of the Americares Free Clinics based in New Canaan, Connecticut). Each served on a volunteer basis, and each put up $1,000 to establish a small financial base. The group met for the first time in January 2002 and began the process of enlisting as members as many of the free clinics nationally as possible. They established a first-year goal of securing membership from at least 100 of the estimated 800 free clinics that existed at that time (a goal that was accomplished). The group was aware that others might criticize the self-appointed basis of the board and perceive the members as attempting to create personal power bases (the same concerns that were raised about the original National Free Clinic Council). So they agreed that they would try to get the association up and running and then rotate others into leadership positions as quickly as possible. The current version of the NAFC's self-description and objectives is reproduced in the accompanying insert.

The National Association of Free Clinics: Self-Description and Objectives

Formed in 2001, the National Association of Free Clinics is a non-profit professional association composed of Free Clinics and State/Regional Free Clinic Associations, working together to support Free Clinics and the people they serve. There are currently over 800 Free Clinics in forty-seven states.

While dozens of organizations across the country work to advocate for the care for the uninsured, Free Clinics have been the primary local community response to actually providing care for those in need. The National Association of Free Clinics is the only organization specifically designed to support and protect the efforts of these local programs on a national basis. Our goal is to unite this diverse group of dedicated organizations into a powerful voice for the uninsured. To accomplish this, the NAFC has established these goals:

- To increase networking among member Free Clinics through electronic media, resource development, and meeting opportunities;
- To monitor and provide input on national legislative and regulatory issues affecting Free Clinics' ability to provide services, and to network and assist state and regional Free Clinic Associations with similar state issues;
- To educate the general public, state and federal leaders and health care industry leaders about the Free Clinic industry and the value that Free Clinics bring to the health care system;
- To develop membership benefits that provide cost-saving opportunities to Free Clinics, and to leverage in-kind donations and gifts:
- To encourage high standards of operations and quality of care;
- To develop national fundraising and resource development opportunities with the goal of passing resources to the local level.

Source: www.nafclinics.org

ISSUES REGARDING THE NAFC

The announcement of the national association met with enthusiasm among many (seventy clinics signed on in the first few months), a wait-and-see attitude among many (waiting to join and to pay dues until they were sure that the national association was really going to survive), and skepticism and concern among others. Those who had concerns about the national association raised four particular issues: (1) whether a national association would truly be able to represent the diversity of approaches embodied in free clinics, (2) the method of appointment of the initial leadership group, (3) the size of the membership fee, and (4) whether or not the association would advocate for particular political positions.

First, even in creating state and regional associations, questions had been raised about the ability of a collective organization to adequately represent the diversity of structures and approaches found in individual clinics. While state associations have been very successful in addressing this issue, it is natural that the issue would also be raised with regard to a national association. In this case, the task for the association would logically be even larger given the number of free clinics in the country and regional and statewide differences—what Tom Rives, MD, medical director of the Friendship House Clinic in Conway, South Carolina, calls their "amazing uniqueness." Some thought that the strong community emphasis of free clinics should be more of a guide for their development than that of a national association.

> My sense is that the viability of our free clinic will depend more on being an integral, indispensable, and consistently effective part of how Virginia delivers health care than as a part of a national organization. Because the needs are so state-specific, in so many cases, free clinics are going to have to identify themselves more with their own locale than with a national organization. (Richard Surrusco, MD, one of the founders of the Bradley Free Clinic, Roanoke, Virginia)

> Creating a national association might be even a little tougher to do than creating a state association because you are not dealing with just one state but with a whole bunch of them. There are regional approaches to things. It might take longer to work everything out. Think how many people this small group of people is working with. (Jeri White, Executive Director, The Community Clinic of High Point, High Point, North Carolina)

For some, however, the idea of a national association has even more appeal because of the diversity of clinics around the country and the fact that medical situations are different from state to state. In this case, a national association could become the one free clinic association that has a global perspective about free clinics and has recognition of their differences as well as commonalities.

I am very positive about the state association and what we are doing to advocate for the rights of the uninsured. . . . The state association helps to put the message out there in advocating for the uninsured; they provide a unified voice. I think in Virginia that we have seen that free clinics have grown. I don't think that we would have been able to do that without a state association. I think no one really understands the plight of the uninsured the way we do. There isn't another medical organization that does what we do. When we talk about universal coverage, we need to have free clinic associations at the table. I have the same enthusiasm for the national association. There should be a force at the state level and at the national level. The needs of the uninsured in Virginia are different than the needs of the uninsured in California. It is a piece of the puzzle that I am not always confident that our policymakers are aware of because most of the people we see are not strong advocates for themselves. Patients come here, and we do know them, so we are able to advocate for them. The national association will be able to paint a new picture of health coverage. (Suzanne Sheridan, Executive Director, Rockbridge Area Free Clinic, Lexington, Virginia)

The formation of state associations and the national association can be a very positive thing. Anytime that you have a group of well-intentioned people sharing information and learning, each doesn't have to reinvent the wheel. Obtaining more funds for clinics would be very important. They can share with Congress information about the potential for free clinics. There is the chance to genuinely educate more people about free clinics. (John Garvin, MD, longtime Board of Directors President and volunteer, Bradley Free Clinic, Roanoke, Virginia)

As it has been at the state and regional level, the issue of regulatory standards has been raised vis-à-vis the national association. Some see the establishment of standards as promoting at least minimal levels (or higher) of quality control, while others oppose such standards because they could detract from the individuality and uniqueness of each clinic.

One of the joys of working in a free clinic is that we are short on bureaucracy. Patients complete just four short papers. The doctors who come here examine the patient, write out progress reports, and maybe write a prescription. . . . They get to actually do some doctoring and not have to write until doomsday about each patient. They like that a lot. . . . There are not a lot of free clinic regulations because clinics are so varied, and they are community-led and community-owned usually by just a scrappy group of people. It would be very hard to regulate that, especially when you don't have a standard type of staff at each clinic. So it is really nice not to be regulated. But regulations can also help a clinic to organize, and so when we do get to the point in the future, and I expect that we will have some type of regulatory body, it may be good for us. (Parker Sparrow, Executive Director, The Free Medical Clinic, Columbia, South Carolina)

As clinics become more known and more recognized and better funded, pressure will increase to standardize and to have regulations that all clinics must follow. But we must resist this pressure to be homogenized because then we lose our greatest strength. It is a difficult thing. Creating standards is a logical next step, but with free clinics, the further that goes, the more it endangers our strength. We must not lose our individuality. (James Beckner, Executive Director, Fan Free Clinic, Richmond, Virginia)

Second, some in the free clinic community have questioned the manner in which the initial leadership board came into being and the fact that there was a leadership board before there was a constituency. Some individuals who have contributed significantly to free health clinics at the state, regional, or national levels were disappointed at not being included in the leadership group and felt that their experiences would have been very helpful to the group.

I believe that you build an organization from the ground up. That was my motive in 1996 [in starting the Free Clinics of the Great Lakes Region]. Our goal was not massive, it was relationship-based, and it was pragmatic. The goal of the FCGLR is to help clinics pragmatically. We are moving toward advocacy, we are moving to develop and grow, but we are doing it one step at a time. I feel that it is essential to start from the ground up. . . . What is the national association doing to build consensus, to build a constituency? I find it difficult to understand why one would establish a national effort and hope to have a national conference without a constituency to invite. It would seem that you start from the ground up, so I was frustrated when the effort was made to identify leaders. How do you define a leader? A big clinic? And a small clinic doesn't have a leader? Clinics in rural areas don't have leaders? I don't think that is true. It was my suggestion that we identify the states in the country for which we have no information with regard to volunteer-based health clinics. And that we each take a couple of states and work very diligently to identify where the free clinics are in these states. Can we make contact? Can we build a relationship and rapport? Engage them? Who knows—they may have the best idea since sliced bread, and no one knows about it. That was put down in a heartbeat that that was a bad idea. I don't know how else you build a constituency other than from the ground up. . . . To say that there isn't a need for some national group, I wouldn't deny that for a minute. But I believe that you build it from the ground up, and you nurture . . . it has to be for the collective good. And, basically, that is where I come from. I am not saying that they aren't working hard and don't have a good intent—I would not say that in a million years. I just feel it is something you build from the ground up and not the top down. (Jane Zwiers, Executive Director, Kalamazoo Free Clinic, and Director, Free Clinics of the Great Lakes Region)

There are still many unknowns about the national association. It is great for one group to do it, but before you call it a national association, you need to branch out and get input from around the country on structure, mission, and composition before saying we are the national association, send us your money. (Randall Rhea, Board of Directors President, Bradley Free Clinic, Roanoke, Virginia)

Group leaders considered formation of a national association as an obvious next step in free clinic development and were frustrated that it had not materialized. The FDA regulations stimulated the sense of urgency that a collective voice at the national level was needed immediately in order to have the legitimacy to negotiate with the FDA to eliminate the new regulations. The group was composed of very dedicated free clinic individuals from, generally speaking, across the United States and especially from areas (such as Virginia and North Carolina) where there was a heavy concentration of free clinics. Each perceived work on the national association to be a significant contribution to the continuing and enhanced development of free clinics, which was seen as being a crucial step in better serving the needs of the uninsured. They intended to do the organizational work and then rotate in new waves of leadership.

> Our vision was to get this thing started, so that we could get some other people involved in leadership roles. Our job was to create the organization, so that more people could come in and make their contributions to it. (Marty Hiller, Executive Director, Free Clinic of Greater Cleveland, Cleveland, Ohio)

Third, in order to develop a sound financial basis, the executive board established a membership fee structure in which the amount of dues was based on the clinic budget. Clinics with larger budgets were asked to pay a larger fee; a typical membership fee was $1,000. For some clinics who wished to join the association, however, this fee level was considered to be prohibitive.

> We have thought about joining the national association. There were dues that we couldn't make. Really, the association would be great. It could offer perks like bulk purchasing. But I think the reason that we decided against it was the fees. We just don't have that kind of money to join an association—that money could be spent on medications. To try to justify that to our patients and then to our board would be difficult. We try to join as many organizations as possible because of the benefits of networking, but when there are fees involved, we just can't. There are several other organizations that we would like to join that could help us, but the fees are just too steep. (Laura Michalski, Director of Clinical Relations, CommunityHealth, Chicago, Illinois)

> I think a national association is a great idea, but the fees to join were based on annual budgets. I could not afford to take the amount of money out of my annual budget to join—it is just cost-prohibitive. I would love to know what is going on nationally. I don't know if it will take off or not. A better idea might be

to form smaller groups like Free Clinics of the Great Lakes and then to have a representative from each of those groups go to the national association. And, if they wanted to have a national conference every year, then anybody could go. The regionals would be better at dealing with particular problems in that area. Many of the people that I have talked to have not been able to afford to join. There is no way that I could justify to the hospital spending that amount of money when we are trying to do so many other things. There are no dues to Indiana or to the Free Clinics of the Great Lakes Region. Our national dues would have been $1,000. (Carla Bice, Executive Director, St. Joseph Health Center, South Bend, Indiana)

There is no exact formula to calculate an ideal level at which a membership fee should be set, and there are competing pressures. On the one hand, the fee should not be so high that interested free clinics are discouraged from joining. On the other hand, the fee needs to be sufficiently high to generate enough funds to put into place the desired programs. For example, to have someone close to the Washington scene who can monitor legislative proposals, make connections with key political officials and government staff members, and be able to testify on a regular basis alone is an expensive proposition. The budget-based membership fee system that was enacted has enabled many free clinics to join and has generated a significant amount of revenue, but has prevented some clinics from being able to join. Recently, the membership fee scale has been recalibrated, so that the fee is now significantly less for most clinics.

The fourth issue related to the founding of the national association is the extent to which the association would take advocacy positions or adopt a political agenda. Some clinic staff expressed concern that the free clinic movement would become more politically focused and less organizationally focused—that attempting to influence policy would have greater priority than strengthening individual clinics and starting new ones. For some, the movement toward formal organization suggests bureaucracy, something they hoped free clinics to be able to avoid. For some, the concern was about the nature of the political agenda that would be adopted.

The good news is that we have enough of a presence to have organized. I think the bad news is that we have enough of a presence to have organized. I see them [the national association leadership group] as a very political group with very definite agendas, and I would hope that the patient population continues to be a priority. By definition, once you have created a political organization, it has to operate politically. Unfortunately, when you do that, you run the risk of forgetting what the original mission is. I think there is risk of alienating some free clinics who don't think they are getting an adequate share of the pie, that the free clinics from the largest catchment areas will have the loudest voice. You have the risk of losing some of the sixties-era-mentality volunteers who perceive this is just another corporate entity in sheep's clothing. They could steer clear, although my experience is that most of them say they will just stay away from that side of it. (Richard Surrusco, MD, one of the founders of the Bradley Free Clinic, Roanoke, Virginia)

Whenever you get organizations coming together, you are going to get some pushing and some pulling, some good and some bad. Most of the state associations offer expertise in grants, funding, indigent drug programs, and education. I see that as being good—I haven't had any bad experiences on the state level. . . . What is coming up now nationally, especially by well-meaning free clinic folks, is a political agenda. And, when you have such a disenfranchised population, I think that the political agenda will tend to radical reform. The desire for radical reform can be the seed of good change, but it can also be disruptive. The real strength of free clinics is the people in the trenches. (Kevin Kelleher, MD, Medical Director, Bradley Free Clinic, Roanoke, Virginia)

This is, of course, a complex issue for the association and one on which it is unlikely that all free clinics will agree. Some members of the executive group and many free clinic people around the country advocate for a national association precisely because of its potential to monitor and speak about proposed legislation and to serve as an important lobbying agent for free clinics and for the uninsured. There is a common sentiment that staff and volunteers in free clinics have a special, experiential expertise in the health and health problems of the uninsured—especially of the working poor. Many see this expertise as providing not only an opportunity but even a responsibility to address their health care needs on a national level.

The qualitative difference between state associations and the national association, for me, is that there will be less of the institutional support focus—that is, tell me how to do something—at the national level when compared to state organizations. The national association has incredible potential for making a difference for free clinics by influencing policy and preventing policies that would harm free clinics. So I believe we at the national level are in a position to speak to access issues because health care is a national issue. What brought us together as a national organization was a public policy matter that could have had a very negative impact on free clinics across the country and their ability to deliver services. It was all about pharmaceuticals. It would not have been an issue for the FDA if a few of us had not made it one. This is why I think the coming together of the national association has a good opportunity of taking hold and evolving and making a difference. We didn't try to start this organization by imagining what it could do and then painting that picture for everyone. We came into being because we said, "If we don't, then this is what is going to happen." And, it has already happened, and we are just trying to catch up with it. There have been a lot of people who have had their eyes opened as a result of it. So I'm sure the national association will be more political than the state associations in terms of its work. It will be to a much higher degree issue-oriented. Health care issues are state- or national-focused. For this reason, the national association has dedicated resources to helping both of those forums come into play. (Marty Hiller, Executive Director, Free Clinic of Greater Cleveland, Cleveland, Ohio)

A national association can't do everything for everybody, but it should be a representative of everyone for a general purpose. Putting together a lobby should be one of its highest priorities—lobbying and being able to make an impact on legislation, to enhance legislation as well as to defeat harmful legislation. . . . It can't simply be a bunch of bleeding heart do-gooders. That is not what an association is. An association must be a business, a hard-core objective operation that is a watchdog for its members in all areas. (Eric Riley, Executive Director, Canton Community Clinic, Canton, Ohio)

This kind of difference of opinion is certainly common in organizational development and growth and especially complex because the various factions are all genuinely devoted to free clinics and to caring for the uninsured.

DEVELOPMENT OF THE NAFC

The issues that have surfaced in forming a national association have demonstrated once again the passion that individuals have for free clinics and the diversity of understandings about them. In the late 1960s and early 1970s, the National Free Clinic Council was a logical and potentially beneficial effort, but it was brought down by internal politics, differences in views about the ultimate goals of free clinics and of the national association, and concerns that some individuals were taking on too much power. The issues with the National Association of Free Clinics have not been altogether different.

But the National Association of Free Clinics (NAFC) is developing an increasingly strong base. The number of free clinics joining the national association continues to grow. Leaders hope that efforts to help free clinics and the patients they serve will convince more and more clinics to want to affiliate. Some of the most visible current efforts are to facilitate networking within and across states; to make clinics aware of publications, Web sites (such as that of the Center for Medicare Advocacy), and resources (such as a Spanish-language medical help telephone number sponsored by the Department of Health and Human Services); to produce materials (such as a new guide to assist free clinics in complying with the HIPAA [Health Insurance Portability and Accountability Act] guidelines on patient privacy); and to strengthen legal protection for individuals who volunteer in free clinics (a national survey is currently underway to obtain information about medical malpractice coverage around the country for free clinic volunteers).

Mark Cruise, executive director of the Virginia Association of Free Clinics and former interim executive director of the National Association of Free

Clinics, summarizes his perspective on the process and development of the NAFC:

> It took a long time and a lot of work to build a consensus as to what the purpose of the Virginia Association of Free Clinics would be and how it would operate and be structured and be governed. I think that same rocky road has manifested itself in the national association. I think it is a function of the diversity of free clinic people and the individuality and independence of free clinics. Clinic people, while being very dedicated to increasing access to health care are very independent-minded and strong-willed and protective of the free clinic concept as they know it. There is even to this day and will be forever a broad diversity of free clinic opinions, backgrounds, and experiences in the free clinic world. And, I think that has contributed to the lack of ability to expeditiously move to the creation of a national free clinic association. . . . Obviously, we are still in the infancy of the organization.
>
> What exacerbates things now more than ever is that you have people in the free clinic world on polar opposites of the political spectrum. I think in the early days free clinics were much more homogenous, at least that's my observation, and now there are some free clinics that are made up by and led by very conservative-minded people and those that are led by very liberal-minded people. They have very different visions about what a national association should be and do.
>
> Where the discussion really gets interesting is where you talk about what the policy agenda should be for the national association. The liberal-minded people would like to see universal health care. The conservative-minded people would object to that. The real challenge of the national association will be how to bring people together, to reach consensus, to build bridges, and to create an organization where people can work together, and maybe agree or disagree about some things, but keep moving forward.

7

Free Health Clinic Staff and Volunteers

I love my job and would not change it for anything. I love coming to work each day. If someone asked what I would most like to be doing, I would say this.

(Laura Michalski, CommunityHealth)

BACKGROUND OF NONPROFIT AGENCIES

I want to tell you about my mother. I came here from Pennsylvania. I worked at the Department of Labor for eleven years. I had a good job, but my mother got sick. She had a stroke, and she died when she was fifty-six years old. My mama died because, being on Medicare, she could not afford her medicines. She would take one medicine one week and a different medicine the following week. Then she tried portioning it out. Her system got so messed up because she was not being maintained with the medications. Eventually, they couldn't do anything for her. They said that, if they did surgery, she would have a heart attack or stroke. So that's why I know what we do here is a very important thing. I have seen in my own family what juggling medicine and not having medicine will do. (Regina Hutchinson, Executive Director, Mercy Medicine Clinic, Florence, South Carolina)

There are more than one million nonprofit organizations in the United States, and together they employ more than ten million people—about 7 percent of the total workforce. By definition, nonprofits advocate for a social cause or provide a community service. They may relate to the promotion of the arts, the provision of human services, education, historical preservation, the environment, politics, and other issues that have stimulated group organization for reasons other than to make a profit.

Many nonprofit organizations must scramble for sufficient funds to support their programs—often operating closer to the margin than public or private sector agencies. Financial support may be dependent on annual pleas to governments at one or more levels, grants from public and private foundations, various fund-raising activities, and appeals to private philanthropists and donors. Even in prosperous economic times, many nonprofits struggle to maintain adequate funding. When the economy is in a downturn, pressure on government funds from all sources increases, and discretionary philanthropic giving by individuals decreases. In the last several years, most donors have required greater accountability of funds spent and more documentation of accomplishment of desired ends. Among the benefits accruing from these greater demands are enhanced short-term and long-term planning, clearer formulation of specific objectives, and more systematic determination of the extent to which objectives are being realized. However, these assessment activities can require a significant amount of time, and that exacerbates time pressures for agencies with limited staff.

Funding pressures are the primary influences on two very important patterns in nonprofits: (1) organizational leaders and staff typically are paid lower salaries than they would make in the private sector, and (2) organizations often make extensive use of volunteers to help sustain the organization. Two of the most important tasks for nonprofit organizations are finding a multiply talented executive willing to spend long hours working for a lower salary than could otherwise be earned and establishing a successful program to recruit, use, and reward volunteers. These pressures can be even greater in free health clinics than in other nonprofits because they provide direct medical care services and because they are volunteer-dependent.

Nonprofits occupy something of an ambiguous position in American society. They are part of neither the government nor the private marketplace. They are structured both formally and informally in a myriad of ways, lines of ownership are not always clearly drawn, their purposes span a wide spectrum, and they receive funding from many different sources (Frumkin 2002). In recent years nonprofits have been the object of political tugs-of-war. For different reasons, they are often embraced by both political liberals and conservatives. The fact that people across the political spectrum see potential in the nonprofit sector speaks to its complicated role within society.

Nonprofits have traditionally shared perspective more with those on the political left, as free clinics did in the late 1960s and early 1970s. Peter Frumkin (2002) identifies three reasons for this pattern. First, individuals willing to work for relatively low salary and to volunteer in social service agencies constitute a group of very dedicated people who want to make a difference and to promote social change. Second, nonprofits have been viewed as an ideal partner to the government, or alternative to the government, that could more effectively address the needs of disadvantaged populations. Third, nonprofits have attracted many individuals because they are successful in mobilizing groups around progressive concerns and issues. All three of these reasons characterize the early free clinic staff members and volunteers.

On the other hand, since the early 1980s, conservatives have been increasingly attracted to nonprofit organizations, although for very different reasons. First, conservatives see nonprofits as an alternative to continued or increased public spending on social programs. Private charity and volunteerism are viewed as appealing alternatives to taxation and public spending. Second, conservatives believe that nonprofits, especially those that are faith-based, are free to do what public agencies are not: to accompany assistance with a moral or spiritual message. Finally, nonprofit organizations may have more flexibility in seeking local solutions to social problems as opposed to a uniform national program (Frumkin 2002). While this orientation does not characterize a large number of free clinic staff members, it is present among some, and it is a perspective held by some volunteers.

FREE HEALTH CLINIC STAFF

In most organizations, large and small, for-profit and not-for-profit, the chief executive is the key figure. In smaller organizations, the chief officer may oversee and even enact most or all of the necessary functions: short-term and long-term planning, budgeting and fund-raising, and human resources management including volunteer coordination, public relations, and data management. This is the pattern in smaller free clinics and even in many of those of moderate size.

As the size of clinics expands, every task becomes larger in scope: there are more funds to be raised; more volunteers to be recruited and trained; larger budgets to be developed and monitored; more patients to be scheduled, examined, and followed up on; and more patient charts to be maintained and filed. The work involved in these tasks becomes greater than what any person can do, and the number of staff members increases. If the executive director of the free clinic does not have a clinical background, an early hire often is a clinical services manager who does—a nurse practitioner or a nurse or a physician. If the executive has a clinical background, the first hire is more likely to be a social worker or case manager or volunteer coordinator. A full-time or part-time office manager or receptionist with clerical skills is an essential early hire. Clinics that include a pharmacy or drug dispensary require a paid worker or volunteer to assume responsibility for that service.

Several free clinics have made the decision to apply for public and private grant money in order to develop specifically focused services. In many cases grantors have been willing to underwrite basic services. This is contrary to the typical pattern but is evidence of the needs that have been documented. In other cases grant money has been used for start-up and at least early maintenance of programs targeted to specific need areas. For example, the Davidson Medical Ministries Clinic in Lexington, North Carolina, has used grants from the Duke Endowment Fund and the Kate B. Reynolds Foundation to establish and maintain a chronic disease clinic one afternoon per week. These grants have enabled the hiring of a part-time physician assistant and a part-time licensed pharmacist to focus on diabetics and hypertensives within a comprehensive medical clinic that closely monitors each patient. At CommunityHealth in Chicago, a physician secured a NIH (National Institutes of Health) grant to develop a patient-friendly software program on diabetes. Patients at the clinic can simply touch the screen to activate eleven different diabetes-related programs (e.g., on the eyes or on the feet or on the importance of exercise), available in both English and Spanish. Someone is always available to show patients how to use the system. Clinics that have secured sizable grants to offer additional services typically have larger staffs because the grants include money for staffing positions.

Whatever the stage of development of a clinic and whatever its scope of services, the executive director is a pivotal figure. Board of directors members, staff members, volunteers, and sometimes patients routinely and without prompting identify the executive director of the clinic as being the indispensable centerpiece of the organization. In many clinics, the executive director has the difficult position of being both the chief administrator and the emotional leader of the clinic. While these tasks require different sets of skills (Nanus and Dobbs 2001), in free clinics, both responsibilities often reside in one individual.

Is there a logical track—a common background—that clinic directors have pursued leading up to their appointment at the clinic? No. Most, but not all, executive directors have had prior experience in the health care sector. Many, but not all, have had prior administrative experience. Several first became attached to the clinic as a volunteer and became so committed to the cause that they later applied for and were selected as the executive director. Many came to the clinic early in their work careers; for others, it was a mid- or late-career move. Many have an educational degree in a health care field; many others do not.

One executive director is a former state hospital association president; another was a trained nurse and stay-at-home mom who worked at the clinic for five years and was then hired as director. One was a licensed practical nurse who became a registered nurse, then earned a bachelor of science degree, began volunteering at the clinic, was eventually hired as director, and now has a master of public administration degree; another was an RN who had worked in community mental health. One director first heard about the clinic in a presentation at her church, after which she became a volunteer before being appointed as director. Prior to being the clinic executive, one director had coordinated volunteers in a nursery school; one had been in the military; one had worked in a variety of community service positions. Others include physicians and nurse practitioners and nurses who wanted to focus on serving low-income persons, a church administrator, a spouse of a pharmacist who had volunteered in a free health clinic, a state legislator, a nursing home administrator, a pharmacist, a hospital administrator, and a community health center director. One director holds a master of education degree from a divinity school; another's educational background is in mining engineering. While a background in medicine or nursing is most common, executive directors represent a wide diversity of educational backgrounds and job experiences.

What then distinguishes free health clinic directors? Organizational skills. An ability to be persuasive and a willingness to ask anyone for anything that would help the clinic. Being as much at ease in working with low-income individuals and families as with health care professionals. An ability to multitask. Perhaps more than anything, an extraordinary passion for serving free clinic patients and an ability to articulate this passion. In conversation after conversation with executive directors and those who work for and with them, it is this dedication, empathy, and wholehearted commitment to free clinic patients that is conveyed.

Several of the clinic directors shared their feelings about their work.

We have the opportunity to change other people's lives, and I love that. Collectively, we really do change people's lives. That never gets old. (Estelle Nichols Avner, Executive Director, Bradley Free Clinic, Roanoke, Virginia)

There are many people out there willing to provide medical care to people who can pay. But you don't see people beating down the doors to provide free health care. They don't know what they are missing. These patients are so appreciative. It is not big money, and it never will be. But there is not a day when I go home that I don't feel like I really helped somebody that would not otherwise have gotten help. I love this population. (Cynthia Moore, Clinic Director, Good Samaritan Clinic, Parkersburg, West Virginia)

I love it here. My position is a great combination of patient care, working as part of a movement in trying to create social change and to improve access to care for people across the city. I also get to do teaching—I love being able to supervise the students who come here. (Randi Abramson, MD, Bread for the City/Zacchaeus Free Clinic, Washington, DC)

My motivation for being here is to make things better for other people. There are huge needs out there. I enjoy the challenges of nonprofit management where you have to take the least and turn it into the most and give people things they didn't think that they could get. That is what drives me. (Sheri Wood, Executive Director, Kansas City Free Health Clinic, Kansas City, Missouri)

I value being in the position of being a voice for silent voices, for those who don't have the ability or have the connections to talk on their own behalf about what it is like not to have access to health care. (Joseph Dunn, Executive Director, Los Angeles Free Clinic, Los Angeles, California)

FREE HEALTH CLINIC VOLUNTEERS

In 2003, according to data compiled by the United States Bureau of Labor Statistics, more than sixty million Americans—almost 30 percent of the population age sixteen and over—engaged in some form of volunteer activity. Volunteers were defined as "persons who did unpaid work (except for expenses) through or for an organization" (see www.bls.gov.cps, 1). Women were somewhat more likely than men to volunteer, and likelihood of volunteering is higher among those with more education and with higher incomes. Rate of volunteering increases through the midforties (thirty-five- to forty-four-year-olds being most likely to volunteer) and tapers off after that (although more than one in five individuals age sixty-five and older continue to volunteer).

Those who volunteer spend on average about an hour per week in volunteer activities (a median of fifty-two hours for the year), and those sixty-five and older volunteer the greatest number of hours (a median of eighty-eight hours per year). About two-thirds of volunteers work for a single organization to which they are dedicated; about 20 percent volunteer for two organizations. The types of organizations for which people are most likely to volunteer are religious (a site for more than one-third of volunteers) and educational and youth-based programs (a site for just under 30 percent). The next most common volunteer sites (though they attract significantly fewer volunteers) are social and community service organizations (just over 10 percent of volunteers) and hospitals or other health organizations (just under 10 percent).

Most volunteers do not engage in activities that overlap with their primary job responsibilities. The most common volunteer activities are fundraising and selling items to raise money; coaching, refereeing, tutoring, or teaching; collecting, preparing, distributing, or serving food; providing information, including being an usher, greeter, or minister; and engaging in general labor. A slight plurality of volunteers became involved after being asked to do so by the organization or by a friend or family member or by an employer, while about 40 percent took the initiative to contact the organization (www.bls.gov.cps).

Volunteering in a Free Health Clinic

Though precise figures are not collected, there may be more than 50,000 individuals in the U.S. who volunteer in free health clinics. Volunteers are drawn from the health professions (e.g., physicians, nurses, dentists, pharmacists, mental health therapists), from education (from health professional schools and from undergraduate and graduate institutions), and from lay sectors throughout society.

There are four key ways that volunteers and volunteering in free health clinics differ from typical patterns: (1) the dependence of clinics on volunteer staffing, (2) the fact that health care professionals use their primary skills in their volunteer work, (3) the fact that a high percentage of volunteers are employed full-time, and (4) the unusual configuration of full-time staff, part-time staff, health care professionals, and lay volunteers working together to provide patient services.

First, free health clinics *depend* on volunteers to provide patient services. In most settings volunteers supplement the work of full-time and part-time staff members. While there are many variations, the most essential tasks in organizations are carried out by paid staff members, decision-making authority resides with the paid staff, and volunteers are used to provide support services. This is not to say that the work of volunteers is unimportant. That is not correct. But volunteers often provide important, nonvital services so that paid staff can fulfill the essential tasks.

However, most free clinics have only a small or relatively small paid staff, which may include only one or a small number of health care professionals, and volunteers carry out necessary and vital activities. For example, the Hollywood Sunset Free Clinic in California has about thirty staff but almost 200 volunteers. The Kalamazoo Free Clinic in Michigan has the equivalent of four and a half full-time paid staff and 350 volunteers. The CommunityHealth Clinic in Chicago has the equivalent of fourteen full-time paid staff members and 350 volunteers. In the year 2000 alone, free health clinics in Virginia served over 42,000 patients and provided more than $31 million in medical care, and they did so with the help of 2,300 volunteer physicians, 900 volunteer nurses, 250 volunteer pharmacists, and 325 voluntary dentists.

This is a profound difference. It dramatically increases the responsibility for securing a sufficient number of volunteers to discharge clinic work, and it requires coordination of clinic activities and record keeping to permit the smooth flow of activities by a variety of providers. Sandy Motley, Director of Davidson Medical Ministries Clinic in Lexington, North Carolina (a clinic with almost 200 volunteers), expresses it this way:

> We are always recruiting volunteers. Working with a largely volunteer staff is like being on a roller-coaster ride. We are either on top with lots of volunteers, or in a valley losing them, or coming back up the other side. I try to use every

opportunity to speak to civic groups, church groups, and community affairs groups. I learned an important message early on; you never stop telling your story. Most people need to hear a message four or five times before they act on it.

The strain of maintaining sufficient volunteers has led some clinics to search for alternative models that permit retention of the spirit of the clinic while making greater use of paid staff. But relying on volunteers permits an extraordinary amount of work to be done at relatively little cost. This "super-efficiency" is a hallmark of free health clinics and a basis for requesting funding from private and public donors. It is an obvious part of the ambience of most clinics.

Second, unlike many volunteer settings, free clinics enable health care volunteers and some lay volunteers to use their job skills in their volunteer activities. Some volunteers prefer activities that enable them to "get away from" normal job tasks. However, many persons especially enjoy utilizing their special talents in the course of volunteering, feel most comfortable in a routine or relatively routine environment, and consider this to be the most effective way for them to make a contribution. In most communities, the free clinic is the only nonprofit organization that provides direct medical services, and many health care professionals see the provision of direct services as the way they can be of most help.

> There is no better place to use my professional skills. I have always enjoyed providing clinical care. When I am in my own office, patients are here because of insurance, and they have a certain level of expectations. All that is important to pay attention to, and it also can be somewhat wearing—keeping up with expectations, demands, schedules, and because you are getting paid, there is not necessarily obvious appreciation. At the free clinic, you really feel like everything you are doing is going above and beyond, which is great. Patients are extraordinarily appreciative, and we have just as much time as we could possibly need with each patient—a very nice thing. (Doug Van Zoeren, MD, former medical director and current board member and volunteer clinician, Washington Free Clinic, Washington, DC)

A third way that volunteering in free health clinics differs from typical volunteering is that many of the volunteers work at full-time jobs. The nation's pool of volunteers draws heavily from those who are retired, are temporarily out of the workforce, or are employed part-time. These individuals often have more available time to volunteer and more flexibility in their schedule. They can be available when an organization most needs help, which is often during the day on weekdays. While they often make use of these groups, free clinics tend to draw more heavily on persons working full-time. This is a testimony to the dedication of these individuals. Many physicians, nurses, other health care professionals, and laypersons work a full day at their job and then go to the clinic (often directly) to volunteer during evening hours. The fact that many clinics offer evening hours is not mere coincidence. Because they often see patients who work during the day and who would not get paid for leaving the job to obtain medical care, evenings are the primary needed time. The small kitchens in many free clinics are more than a luxury; they provide food for volunteers who go directly from work to clinic.

Clinics that also offer daytime hours or do so exclusively are more likely to have some paid health care professionals and to use retired health care and lay volunteers. Clinics that use retired physicians are uniform in their praise. They see them as individuals who want to remain productive and whose volunteering tends to be motivated largely by a desire to serve others. Even in these clinics, however, it is not unusual to find volunteers who work full-time and volunteer in the clinic on their day off.

Many full-time health care professionals say that they volunteer at free clinics because they are able to practice medicine the way they would prefer:

We have a lot of volunteer physicians who battle managed care all day, and they say that they gladly volunteer for the free clinic for three hours at night because there are no administrative hassles, no managed care, no preauthorization, just "take care of the patients and feel better about it." (Richard Seymour, administrator, Haight-Ashbury Free Clinics, San Francisco, California)

One of our volunteer physicians comes here because she gets to practice the art of medicine. She doesn't have to worry about the diagnostic code, whether or not the insurance company is going to pay for this or that test, what test she has to run first in order to be sure that the insurance company will pay for the second test. She doesn't have to worry about any of that. She comes here because she gets to practice the art of medicine which she was trained to practice. (James Beckner, Executive Director, Fan Free Clinic, Richmond, Virginia)

For whatever reason clinicians first volunteer here, I know why they come back. Everybody pretty much says the same thing. Whether it is the pharmacist, the nurse, the physician, it doesn't matter, everybody may walk in here at 6:00 on a Thursday night and be really tired from the day's work. They may be thinking, "if I could just go home, how many patients do we have?" But, by the time they walk away, they all say the same thing—it was a great evening and that they really helped these people. (Cynthia Moore, Clinic Director, Good Samaritan Clinic, Parkersburg, West Virginia)

Fourth, one can walk into almost any free clinic at any time and find a wide assortment of paid staff, health care professionals, and lay volunteers from all walks of life. Some volunteer health care professionals feel most comfortable in their white coat, but many discard it at the clinic. Some physicians think it most appropriate at the clinic to be referred to as Doctor So-and-so, but many use only a first name. In almost all clinics, however, all volunteers work side by side without attention to the usual status gradations. When clinics are busy, they tend to be very busy, and attention is focused on patients and patient care.

Laura Michalski, director of clinic relations at the CommunityHealth Clinic in Chicago, describes the atmosphere that permeates her clinic as like that of a family. Volunteers are there because they want to be part of this community service and because they enjoy working together. She describes a common scene in which a volunteer physician works closely with a volunteer high school student who is serving as an interpreter for the patient. Several directors refer to the respect that health care professional and lay volunteers have for each other while they provide patient services. Observing clinic sessions, it is easy to see the palpable energy that exists during clinic hours and genuine feelings of working together to best take care of patients.

Staff and Volunteer Motivations

There is an extensive scholarly literature that reports on the motivations that prompt individuals to become volunteers. Given the extremely hectic pace of life that most persons experience and the many competing demands for time, there must be significant reasons for an individual to make a volunteer commitment. Free clinic volunteers identify six primary motivations underlying their commitment: (1) a belief in the importance of providing health care to all persons, (2) a sense of personal accomplishment and fulfillment from working at the clinic, (3) personal growth and learning experiences, (4) friendships and sense of bonding with others at the clinic, (5) faith-based or spirit-based reasons, and (6) the importance of "giving something back" to the community. This section elaborates on these motivations and illustrates them in the words of free clinic volunteers.

The Importance of Providing Health Care to All Persons

Perhaps the most important reason that people volunteer is to contribute to a cause in which they really believe. Many Americans believe that all persons in this country should have accessible health care services and that no one should have to experience health-related pain and suffering because they cannot pay for private medical care. The United States guarantees access to public education for all persons—it has deemed formal education to be so important that public funds are committed to ensuring available schools and teachers for all children. Although access to health care is an issue about which many persons are very concerned, no similar commitment has been forthcoming. The United States is alone among modern countries in the world in failing to make this commitment.

The basis for working at or volunteering in a free health clinic for many health care professionals and many lay volunteers is a genuine belief in this cause. However, this "cause" is defined in different ways by different individuals and different clinics. All of the early free clinics and many contemporary clinics share a commitment to having available health care for all persons whatever their circumstances and whatever their financial condition. These clinics hold the view that health care is a "right"—not just a privilege—and that the government has an unfulfilled responsibility to guarantee access to health care for all. Free clinics are viewed as agencies that have stepped in to help fill the need because the government has failed to do so. David Smith, MD, from the Haight-Ashbury Free Clinics and others articulate this position:

Our mission, philosophy, and delivery of care is for the uninsured and for those who have been rejected by the mainstream of society; our motto is that health care is a right, not a privilege. The United States is the only industrialized country in the world that does not have some form of national health insurance or a safety net. And that philosophy that came out of the sixties is very much a part of the mainstream debate as it hits the elderly, dot.coms and so many others who have gotten laid off. Every time that you are exposed to what it is like when you don't have health insurance and access to primary care, you become a health care activist.

I am concerned about health care for people and the fact that our government does not guarantee it. I have felt that something needed to be done for the poor and even for the middle class, which is having a rough time today with the cost of medical care. I don't think free clinics are the answer to medical care, but it is a stopgap measure, and until something else comes along, we just have to make this work. (Franklin Bacon, volunteer, Charlottesville Free Clinic, Charlottesville, Virginia)

In the last few years, as a health care provider, I have been increasingly disillusioned. I have been a nurse for thirty years, and there seems to be an increase in the number of health care providers who reach a point with a patient and then not provide additional services. Recently, we had a patient here who had been diagnosed with cancer, and it was metastasized. She was going to need a lot of medical care, and her provider referred her to us. He said that he could no longer see her because she could not pay. I was just flabbergasted. I have always thought that there was some sort of obligation to treat patients regardless of finances—that is something that makes health care providers who they are. In the past, we were always there for people who couldn't pay just like we were always there for people who could pay. And, in my mind anyway, there is a social responsibility in every community to make sure that people who are well off can take care of their community. And, in the last several years, I have seen this dwindling desire to help others. As a taxpayer, I can understand the issues on one level, but that doesn't change the fact that there are people out there who don't have the capacity to access the care system. (Terri Bliziotes, Clinical Program Coordinator, West Virginia Health Right, Charleston, West Virginia)

The motivation of our volunteers? They believe that health care ought to be a right. Truly. They are not looking for any money, they are not looking for certificates, they truly believe that health care is a right and that there is a genuine need. (Tacy Padua, Executive Director, Hollywood Sunset Free Clinic, Los Angeles, California)

For me, I so strongly believe that health care is a basic human right like food, clothing, and shelter. That philosophy is so deeply embedded in who I am that I can't even imagine health care for reimbursement. (Susan Mandel, MD, Medical Director, Los Angeles Free Clinic, Los Angeles, California)

Not all free clinic staff and volunteers would agree on the best way to provide care for everyone. The fact that nonprofit organizations today appeal to both the Left and the Right is perfectly illustrated in free health clinics. Many free clinic staff members, but not all, around the country believe that the government should guarantee available health care for all persons. This is especially the case in free clinics that were created in the early years, free clinics in large cities, and free clinics on the West Coast. Volunteers in free clinics, however, tend to come from a variety of political positions. Some support the free clinic for the reasons that nonprofits have traditionally been more tied to liberal ideology. But others' support of free clinics is more aligned with conservative ideology.

How do free clinics handle this situation? Certainly, there is not a single, uniform response. But most free clinics are very careful to keep their focus on the patients. As long as staff and volunteers provide high-quality, compassionate care for patients, most free clinics pay no attention to their political ideology. In fact, most clinics want to draw support from across the political spectrum, and they rely on such support to have sufficient volunteers and financial contributions.

Quite frankly, we run from political discussions as fast as we can. I suspect that our volunteers are all over the map, so at this agency, we have decided not to take any political stands. I actually was a lobbyist in another life, so I am used to politics, and I am used to telling people what I think and how I would like to see things done. This job has really made me reverse that type of thinking, at least for this job. It is hard for me not to express my personal politics, but we found out very early that our supporters are all over the map, that they weren't of a particular political persuasion. One of our doctors recently wrote a letter to the newspaper that stirred a lot of discussion about a call for universal health care. Some of it was from other doctors who are a part of this program who said that is not what they want. We received one of [the first] President Bush's "points of light." There are some providers in our program who see that as a Republican thing—that communities take care of their own without government intervention, that communities can do it best at the grassroots level, and that government money isn't the answer to everything. So that is why they are part of it. We have those two extremes among our volunteers, and because we don't want to alienate any of those people from our program, we don't take a stand. What we do take a stand on is that programs like ours are not the ultimate answer for the uninsured in the community, but we don't lead the way in promoting how change should occur. (Barb Tylenda, Executive Director, Health Care Network, Inc., Racine, Wisconsin)

There are some physicians who volunteer here who would not support universal coverage. They feel, as physicians, they should volunteer at the clinic as opposed to supporting universal coverage. But I would say they are in the minority. I would venture a guess that, whether they are Democrats or Republicans, most have an ideology that would support universal health coverage. We are really talking about free clinics responding to a local human need. It is not as much ideology as it is in your face. As a result, it appeals to people, not politics. I have been a volunteer for, I don't know, I probably started volunteering when I was fourteen years old, and I have never stopped. I have never been involved in an organization that is so broad-based, community-wise. The people who come and help at the clinic come from all walks of life. . . . When I came on the board of directors here and looked at our list of supporters, there were probably an equal number of Democrats and Republicans. (Carol McHaley, Executive Director, DuPage Community Clinic, Wheaton, Illinois)

One of the wonderful things is, we don't go there [political beliefs of volunteers], because that is not important in what we do. I think if we ask that question, we would get very different answers. We focus on the needs of the patients. (Suzanne Sheridan, Rockbridge Area Free Clinic, Lexington, Virginia)

The political ideology of staff and volunteers? Our paid staff are socially liberal. I don't know about volunteers—they are probably a broad representation of political ideology. We would probably be hard-pressed to find any far-right religious conservatives. There is probably a hefty chunk on the liberal side. But this would not be as true for clinics that have started since the mid- to late-1980s. They tend to be more conservative, more apt to be of Christian religious sentiment. . . . There are some very real cultural differences of older clinics and newer clinics. (James Beckner, Fan Free Clinic, Richmond, Virginia)

Personal Accomplishment and Fulfillment

Many free clinic volunteers experience a profound sense of personal fulfillment and accomplishment from their work. Even though they typically spend far less time in the clinic each week or each month than do staff members, volunteers almost universally report this keen sense of fulfillment.

Many volunteer coordinators recognize that the quickest way to lose volunteers is to put them in a situation in which they do not feel needed, in which there are not sufficient tasks to keep them busy, and in which there is an absence of a feeling of making a legitimate contribution. For most persons, life is simply too busy to donate hours to an unneeded activity.

No volunteer site—even free health clinics—is foolproof. Poorly organized volunteer programs with inadequate scheduling and schedule mix-ups, too much downtime, feelings of being taken advantage of, and inadequate support and appreciation typically fail regardless of the nature of the setting. However, given a well-structured program for volunteers, free clinics offer opportunities for tremendously fulfilling volunteer work. In whatever way a volunteer is used—providing direct care services, filling a prescription, taking a social or medical history, making patients feel as comfortable as possible, answering the telephone and making appointments, and others—there is a routine feeling that something has been achieved, that people's lives have been made to feel better due to the efforts of the staff and volunteers. Few people would not be touched by being in a position to affect others so meaningfully and so positively.

Free health clinic staff and volunteers are very articulate about this sense of personal accomplishment. One volunteer physician, a family practice physician and former medical director of the free clinic, recalled a patient story to illustrate his feelings about volunteering at the clinic.

A nineteen-year-old woman came to us from a neighboring state. She had a three-year-old who was crying on the exam table. She was getting away from a relationship in which she had been terribly physically abused. The only way that she could get away was to run away. She arrived here with no resources, but she was trying to do her best with her son. She had not been well prepared for parenthood to begin with, and now she was stuck in a town with a sick child and in which she didn't know anyone. We helped the child, and we asked if we could help her. When you see that kind of patient, you stop and take the time. We hooked her up to all kinds of resources—shelter, community services, child care services. In that young woman's life, the contact with the free clinic was a miracle. It may have been way more than anything that had ever happened to her in her life. Gosh . . . to be part of miracles. The whole free clinic seems to be a miracle.

This is the best job that I have ever had. I come to work every day knowing that I can help someone who has less than I do or is less fortunate. No matter how bad the day is, I still leave with a good feeling knowing that in some way, I am making a difference in their lives and in the quality of care that they are receiving. (Robin Roberson, Office Manager, Community Free Clinic, Hagerstown, Maryland)

Why do I work here? I see the need. It is the need. It is about the people who are a little bit less fortunate than you are. When a patient comes in and they have been down and out, and you talk with them for a while, they will often say how much they have been helped. It does your heart good. I like the work that I do, and their response makes it special. (Verle Harrelson, Administrative Assistant, Free Medical Clinic, Columbia, South Carolina)

The clinic keeps people alive. Each year, we dispense or provide access to about $250,000 worth of medicines to our patients. Those patients would do completely without most of the time if not for us. So a lot of them are having a slow death without their medications. We make a huge difference for them, adding quality and quantity to their lives. Most people would be without care and were without care before we were here. (Sandra Drury, Executive Director, Free Clinic of Reidsville and Vicinity, Reidsville, North Carolina)

People are my passion, and I am more effective with people than with things. I found this out when I was a hospice volunteer and then when I became a staff member and then went to nursing school. After my first year of nursing, I worked in medsurg at Hopkins, and I was very frustrated by having to do so much with things. I decided that would be my last experience doing that. Then, I got into community work in a very poor area in Baltimore when I was a manager of a hypertension study. And I loved it. . . . I just loved it. I loved the teaching. I loved having people learn how to take care of themselves, and it really did something to me. Then, I was in another job in East Baltimore when this opportunity [at the free clinic] came along. Though I liked what I was doing, I realized this is where I wanted to be . . . being able to see a smile on a person's face and to know that I helped to make it happen. (Anne Barker, Nurse Clinic Manager, Health Alliance for Patients in Need, Columbia, Maryland)

For many people when they are preparing for death, their greatest fear is whether their life has been worth living. When I ask if I have made any mark on life, I think that I have had the opportunity to be a participant in something that really did change people's lives. It provided a service for somebody that was really needed. (Vic Skaff, DDS, volunteer and cofounder of the dental clinic, Bradley Free Clinic, Roanoke, Virginia)

I enjoy being a small part of helping to meet the need. At the end of the day, I feel good because I have helped to make others' lives a little easier; I have genuinely listened to them; and I have helped to connect them to needed resources. (Carolyn Wilcoxen, Administrative Assistant and Financial Secretary, Good Samaritan Clinic, Parkersburg, West Virginia)

There is so much need, and we are really helping. We have elderly people who cannot work, pregnant teenagers who were kicked out of the house, and so many more. We make such a huge difference in people's lives. (Rachel Reiner-Good, volunteer and granddaughter of the founder—Walt Reiner—Hilltop Health Center, Valparaiso, Indiana)

My grandmother (a patient of the founder of the clinic) shared with me a love for all people. Our patients without insurance often suffer needlessly. . . . Last night, we had a patient who was in tears because he had gotten to this point in his life. We reassured him that we were not judging him, that we were glad that he came, and we were able to give him the care that he needs. (Pamela Idol, RN, Medical/Dental Coordinator, Davidson Medical Ministries Clinic, Lexington, North Carolina)

I always wanted to be a nurse to take care of people who had problems. When I got into nursing and was working in a hospital, I found that most of my focus was taking care of the mandates from regulatory agencies, and there was not a whole lot of room for any creativity. What JACHO [the Joint Accrediting Commission on Hospitals] says, you have to do. If it doesn't necessarily work for your community, or for your population, too bad, it has to meet the criteria for the organization to be certified. The other thing is that any time you tried to do anything creative in a hospital or clinic that was receiving any outside funds or oversight, you sort of got put under the thumb. Here, there are just a couple of key guiding principles. The first is, "Do right by the patient." So it puts all of your energy every day into the care of the patient. This gives me an opportunity to expand my wings, to grow, to be creative, whereas every other place it had to be done in a particular way, and it didn't always make any difference whether it was good for the patient or not. The patients here get the best care that I have seen anywhere. (Terri Bliziotes, Clinical Program Coordinator, West Virginia Health Right, Charleston, West Virginia)

Some of the executive directors, volunteer coordinators, and other staff members have observed the reactions—and sometimes surprise—that volunteers have after their initial experience at the clinic.

When the volunteers come here, they are always amazed at the kind of situations that our patients are in. They just don't have the money for insurance. You can't just treat patients, you have to consider the environment in which they live. When our volunteers walk out of here, they just have such a sense of fulfillment because of what they have been able to do. (Cynthia Moore, Clinic Director, Good Samaritan Clinic, Parkersburg, West Virginia)

Two physicians with longtime service to a free health clinic view the sense of fulfillment that volunteers have at clinics as a primary means for attracting additional volunteers.

I feel good about the two hours that I spend there each time that I volunteer. What is going to drive the guy back—because it is a good idea? I don't think so—it is because of the way that participating there makes you feel. And, if you can make people feel good about what they do, they will do it again, and they will tell other people, and they will start doing it, so you have a gradual, exponential increase in support. (John "Lucky" Garvin, MD, longtime medical director and Board President, Bradley Free Clinic, Roanoke, Virginia)

When I talk to potential physician volunteers, I liken practicing at the clinic to the good old days of being a doctor—when you work just for the sake of making someone better, and no one gave you a dime. All of us in private offices have some degree of concern about those who are unable to pay for services. We can say fine, we can provide it in a different way. I have always looked at it as there has to be a safety net, and Friendship House is it. (Tom Rives, longtime medical director and clinical volunteer, Friendship House, Conway, South Carolina)

Finally, Jack McConnell, executive director of the Volunteers in Medicine Clinic in Hilton Head Island, South Carolina and one of the genuine spiritual leaders of free health clinics, shared these comments:

In today's hustle and bustle, we don't take time to allow relationships to happen. And they are worth far more than money. If we tried to stack up enough money to pay all the people who work at free clinics, they wouldn't want it. They would rather have the joy—the deep personal fulfillment.

Personal Growth

Many staff members and volunteers consider opportunities to learn, to have new experiences, and to grow personally as being important benefits of their free clinic work. Free clinics—with their focus on providing needed medical services to patients who would otherwise go without them, with their emphasis on treating each patient with dignity and respect, with their commitment to bringing together diverse services needed by patients, with their reliance on volunteers to provide many of the services—are especially configured to enable feelings of personal growth.

Sairah Husain, who leads the Information and Referral Collective at the Berkeley Free Clinic (working fifteen hours per week and volunteering an additional fifteen hours per week), describes the clinic volunteers as being a very diverse group but including many individuals who are at a transition point in their life—undergraduate students, graduate students, people deciding on a first career or a midcareer transition, people entering retirement. All of these people enjoy learning from each other:

It is really great because of the people you work with, because you get to really know them. They become a type of family, and you also learn a lot from their experiences, because everybody is from a different walk in life, bringing in a different background of where they grew up and what they are doing right now. You really learn a lot from each other. . . . There is always something new to learn. I really enjoy doing information and resource work. You come across so many interesting questions. It feels good to provide a service to someone who is not going to get it anywhere else and to provide it in a way that really makes a difference to them. You learn something new every single day.

Ann Basart, also a Berkeley Free Clinic volunteer, echoes these sentiments:

> Volunteering here is difficult and it is rewarding because it is difficult. I am learn-
> ing a lot, and I like that, but the issues are more complex and more complicated
> and more involved than I had thought. I knew that the national health care
> scene was sort of a disaster, and now I am realizing it even more deeply. I never
> had really worked directly with people who need this kind of facility. I had seen
> them from a distance but had never gotten involved with them. I can see that
> even though we cannot help them enough, there is something that we can do
> to help. It is not full of glory, it is not easy, it is sometimes difficult for me.

Jean Lee, executive director of the Free Medical Clinic of Northern Shenandoah Valley in Winchester, Virginia, enjoys the special configuration of challenges and opportunities of directing a free health clinic in a small community.

> The clinic gives me an opportunity to be a problem solver, to manage my own
> time, to engage in social activism, to promote justice, to have a diversity of chal-
> lenges, to try to pull together a variety of resources, and to try to get others to
> do what they can to help.

Many directors and other staff and volunteers appreciate the fact that free
clinics are never boring and that no two days are alike. The challenges of getting a free clinic to work and to continue to work day after day are an en-
joyable aspect of being associated with a clinic, that "every day when you
walk in, you know that you don't know what new challenges will occur that
day" (Virginia Garza Halstead, Hollywood Sunset Free Clinic, Hollywood,
California). Like many staff and volunteers, Janet Arenas, who works at the
front desk and teaches diabetes classes at CommunityHealth in Chicago and
is studying nutrition, consciously thinks about all that she is learning from
the patients. The clinic offers a real-world setting that often illustrates and
sometimes challenges textbook knowledge.

Communities with a medical school, like Charlottesville, Virginia; Chapel
Hill, North Carolina; and Washington, D.C., often draw upon medical students and residents as clinic volunteers and sometimes use current physicians or those who have retired from the medical school. Most communities
with a college or university use undergraduate student interns or volunteers
who may see their experience as relating to a major in sociology, psychol-
ogy, premed, prenursing, and other fields. Working at the free clinic adds to
the learning process, often exposing students to situations where medical
problems have not received prompt attention and to situations in which the
living environment is clearly contributing to health problems. Rick Seymour
of the Haight-Ashbury Free Clinics says: "One of the functions that free clinics serve is providing training in community medicine for doctors and health
officials who have then moved on into medical care systems and have taken
some of these ideals and concepts with them."

Using residents and medical students requires an additional supervisory level, but one that is often enjoyed. Sandra Clark, medical director for the Robert Nixon Medical Clinic in Chapel Hill, North Carolina, a clinic that primarily serves the homeless, comments on her own responsibilities in this area:

> I certainly value the relationship that I have with the patients and with the volunteers. I enjoy the mentoring process and working with the student coordinators and mentoring them through something that can be very stressful when they see someone who is in very bad shape. It is rewarding to be able to go through the system with them and with the special problems that homeless people have and to help them see a new perspective on homeless patients.

> In addition to serving the poor we are committed to see things flourish in the end for everyone. This is an education and advocacy group at its center . . . it is like a movement to really better the world. How do you prevent things? It is by advocating and educating other people. . . . We have a lot of new young people entering business. If they do not understand social justice, then everything is just a money issue. We have a lot of schools and organizations that come in here to learn about the poor and about social justice. (John Bartolome, St. Anthony Free Medical Clinic, San Francisco, California)

Friendship and Sense of Bonding

Most people enjoy and want personal ties with others, but, given the seemingly constant pressures on their time and energy, it is not always easy to develop and maintain these relationships. Large cities often offer a more impersonal environment in which connecting can be difficult, and small cities and towns may offer fewer social opportunities for meeting others of similar age and interests. Social psychologists report that many individuals long for the idealized version of a tight-knit family, but families now are smaller, more spread out geographically, busier, and often broken apart.

On some occasions, individuals come together with a shared purpose, similar values, a positive sense of social contribution, and feelings of banding together to take on what is an enormous and very challenging task. These are situations that foster the development of close personal ties, a feeling of "family" and camaraderie, and meaningful bonding. Free health clinics often develop in just this way, and it is very common for staff and volunteers to talk about a very special atmosphere that exists among clinic personnel.

> The volunteers here feel very much like a family . . . like a community working toward a very important goal. (Diana Shapiro, Peer Counseling Collective member, Berkeley Free Clinic, Berkeley, California)

We have a wonderful staff and volunteers. We do have fun. We are silly, we laugh, and we have good times even outside the office. The doctors are caring, they want to be here. We all want to be here. (Carol McHaley, Executive Director, DuPage Community Clinic, Wheaton, Illinois)

Everyone here has a type of missionary zeal for helping our patients. People who work in places like this are single-minded. The only goal is to help patients. There is no infighting. It is a great atmosphere because everyone works together. (Alvita Nathaniel, nurse practitioner and one of the founding directors, Mercer Health Right, Bluefield, West Virginia)

For me I stay at the clinic for two reasons: I really do enjoy working with our patient population. Working here has given me a lot of insight into people suffering from addictions and has enabled me to provide them far better service than I was capable of providing. Also, I really enjoy the fact that patients get excellent, compassionate care, and in many other settings where I have worked, they have gotten excellent technical care but not compassionate care. Here you see a really fine balance with our multidisciplinary team approach that provides this type of care. We have the opportunity to interact with physicians, psychiatrists, pharmacists, and counseling staff. We have an excellent multidisciplinary way of treating each one of our patients. They get outstanding care and respect from people in all of those disciplines. Seeing all of that and developing a real love and respect for my coworkers as well is why I have stayed here so long. (Diana Amodia, MD, Haight-Ashbury Free Clinics, San Francisco, California)

Faith-Based or Spirit-Based Reasons

Some volunteers in free clinics are motivated to participate by a sense of religious duty or from spirit-based grounds. These individuals come from many different religious faiths. Even in clinics that are primarily faith-based, volunteers often represent a wide range of religious belief systems. Sociological research has discovered a complex relationship between religious involvement and volunteering. Much research has found that, in general, individuals who participate in religious organizations are more likely to engage in volunteer activities. This influence has been traced to factors such as a greater likelihood of interpreting volunteer service as religious duty, to the development of social networks within the religious group that may lead to a stronger sense of community, and to more personal requests for volunteer involvement. Recent research has discovered, however, that the effect of religion on volunteering varies with the type of volunteer activity. For Catholics and mainline Protestant denominations, religion is related to increased community volunteering. For conservative Protestant denominations, religious attendance is related to greater likelihood of church-related volunteer activity but not to community volunteering. Research has now discovered that different types of religious involvement (for example, attendance and beliefs) may impact volunteering differently (Lam 2002; Becker and Dhingra 2001; Wuthnow 1999; Wilson and Janoski 1995).

In some cases, free clinic staff and volunteers see their work at the clinic as related to or inspired in general by their religious beliefs or spiritual beliefs. In other cases commitment to clinic work is viewed as a response to a particular religious passage. For example, Macon Baird, executive director of the Open Door Clinic of Alamance County in Burlington, North Carolina, says that he and many of the volunteers at his clinic are very much guided by the biblical passage "to those to whom much is given, much is required." Some clinic staff and volunteers report a sense of "calling" to be at the free clinic.

Many clinic directors describe the motivation of their volunteers as being "faith-based" or "spirit-based" rather than being based in a particular religious organization or belief system. They acknowledge the considerable contributions (both in terms of volunteer time and financial contributions) from a variety of religious bodies. Carol McHaley, executive director of the DuPage Community Clinic in Wheaton, Illinois, characterizes almost all of its volunteers as being "spirit-based" rather than "church-based." The clinic has a close connection with local Methodist churches, Episcopal churches, the Catholic diocese, and the Jewish synagogue. Carla Bice, executive director of St. Joseph Health Center in South Bend, Indiana, describes her volunteers similarly by saying, "Most of our volunteers are faith-based, but not all are of the same faith." Glenn Pierce, executive director of the Asheville-Buncombe Community Christian Ministries Clinic, reports that many of his volunteers "come out of their own Christian witness mission," but that many of the clinic's volunteers "come from their own sense of humanity."

Church-based or faith-based clinics also make a determination of the role that religion plays within the clinic. One of the clinics visited for this study was started by Pastor Keith Goretzka and some congregational members of the First Baptist Church of North Charleston (South Carolina), and the clinic is located within the church. The establishment of the clinic and the acceptance of financial responsibility for it raised questions among church members. Is this a legitimate form of Christian ministry? Is this an appropriate way to use church funds? Would there be security concerns with strangers (that is, clinic patients) coming into the clinic? Would the clinic focus on providing medical care or would there also be volunteers present to discuss religious needs? Pastor Goretzka's message to the congregation focused on scriptural interpretation.

On one side of our church, you will see a scripture from Matthew's gospel on our positive responsibility to provide for the material and physical needs of those who live in the community. I try to remind the congregation that Jesus had a ministry of teaching, preaching, and healing. The message is one of compassion and mercy for those who suffer, particularly for those who cannot provide for their own needs, which is the case here in medical care.

Judy Dillow, who is the director of the Health Care Ministry for the Charleston Baptist Association and the director of this medical clinic and a separate dental clinic, describes the evangelical mission that is part of the clinic.

> This is an evangelical clinic, and our mission is evangelical. Because we are so small, we do not have the resources that some of the larger clinics have, but we offer the hope of Jesus Christ. We are not going to cure all of these people. All we can do is love them in the name of Jesus. That does not mean that we hit them over the head with Bibles, but we do acknowledge spiritual needs as well as physical needs.

The Free Medical Clinic in Columbia, South Carolina, started as the brainchild of a minister, Reverend Bill Bouknight, of the United Methodist Church. As such, the clinic was founded as a faith-based organization, and board members, staff, and volunteers have often discussed exactly what that means. At one point, there was discussion of putting Bibles in the clinic lobby, but that idea was rejected on the basis that the clinic sees patients of many different religious backgrounds—Christians, Jews, Muslims, Hindus, and others. Supporting churches agreed that this was not necessary for the clinic to be serving its mission. A second issue that surfaced was the idea of conducting a prayer before clinic sessions. Parker Sparrow, executive director of the clinic, described the issue this way:

> There has been some discussion of "do we pray or not before clinic sessions?" Certainly, I think that everybody on our staff and our volunteers, or at least most of them, have an active spiritual life. But we chose not to pray as a group before clinic sessions. We decided not to do that because of the amount of diversity that we see in nationalities and religions. I think that religious tolerance, especially with what we are seeing today on the news [the interview was conducted on September 11, 2001] is more important than ever, and though I feel very strongly about the way that I worship, I want everybody that comes around me to have that same freedom. Most of our staff is Christian, our part-time pharmacy director is Jewish and very involved in her synagogue, and our new clinical director is Muslim. I feel strongly about what we are doing here, and I value this diversity.

John Bartolome of St. Anthony Free Medical Clinic in San Francisco describes the ecumenical approach of that faith-based clinic in similar terms:

> When I came here, our statement of values was very grounding to read. I said, "Wow, this is really what I am looking for . . . an organization that is flexible, open, and that is in real solidarity with the poor and really puts its energy into working for the poor." I wasn't sure what I was going to be in for because it was my first Catholic organization. So I was a little apprehensive. But when I came here, I found that it is very ecumenical in its approach, very welcoming of any person in any walk of life.

Wanting to Give Something Back

While modern societies have no shortage of individuals who focus on self and close intimates, there are many others for whom making a contribution to other people or to the wider society is extremely important. This orientation may be faith-based or rooted in more secular grounds. It may be a value that was instilled while growing up, it may have developed during service learning projects in high school or college, or it may have developed later in life. It may be based on a specific notion of reciprocating for one's own opportunities or good fortune, or it may be more generalized. Whatever its origin, many individuals have a clear sense of obligation, or at least an intense desire, to give some of their time, energy, money, and talent to others less fortunate. This orientation is common among free clinic volunteers.

Sandy Motley, executive director of Davidson Medical Ministries Clinic in Lexington, North Carolina, believes her volunteers are motivated by many factors, including social conscience. Many simply believe that they have a social responsibility to reach out and help. Others interviewed also reflected on this motivation.

> I think the motivation of most of my colleagues is one of gratitude, of being able to give back something to the community, and of having received so much. I think the motivation for volunteering at the free clinic is, "I am glad that this is here, and it is a way for me to say thank you." Physicians in general are very grateful for the position they have arrived at in society and appreciate the opportunity to be able to give something back. (Richard Surrusco, MD, volunteer, Bradley Free Clinic, Roanoke, Virginia)

> I have a strong sense of duty to issues larger than myself and a commitment to the clinic. Having been very poor myself at one point, it is easy to have a commitment to our patients. We recognize that the clinic is not making a huge dent in the total needs in society, but we are making a big difference in some people's lives. You do not have to save the world to make a difference in someone's life. (David Kroman, volunteer, Berkeley Free Clinic, Berkeley, California)

> Why do people volunteer here? I just flashed on what many people told me when they became members of the board—that they want to give something back, and they are picking and choosing what they want to give back. I think, in speaking for the receptionists, since I worked there so long, it is people who like to work face to face with people, and make them feel comfortable coming to a free clinic. In the reception area, we are the ones who deal with people's frustrations, not being able to get through on the phone, not being able to get to a private doctor, getting the runaround from county clinics. We set the tone for the clinic—that is a very important job and a very meaningful way to give back. (Frances Helfman, board member, staff member, and volunteer, Los Angeles Free Clinic, Los Angeles, California)

8

Patient Responses and Outcomes

I can't believe that people cared enough to do this for us.

(A free clinic patient)

ATTITUDES OF FREE CLINIC PATIENTS

In the early days of the operation of the clinic essentially all of the patients approached the clinic with apprehension and skepticism. They were distrustful and unsure of us. It was certainly understandable. They had been misled so often that there was no reason to trust. Some told me of their skepticism. They felt the idea of a free medical clinic was a trick that was being played on them. Free health care appeared too good to be true. One could see the lack of trust in their faces when they entered the clinic. They entered hesitantly, seldom looking at you, speaking so softly that it was difficult to hear what they were saying. Even their posture suggested a lack of trust. They stood sideways to you, as if they were in a position to turn and walk away if need be.

[Today] they walk in with a confidence and assurance they will not only receive health care but be embraced in an atmosphere of caring and concern for them as individuals. Their whole demeanor suggests they know they are welcomed and belong here. (McConnell 1998, 95)

What is it like to be a patient at a free health clinic—to know that you and members of your family have gone without needed medical care—to acknowledge that you do not have the resources to obtain private medical care—to call the free clinic to find out about seeing a medical provider—to drive or take public transportation or walk to the clinic—to stand in line or sit in a waiting area with other individuals who are in a similar situation—(in

155

some cases) to give information to someone determining if you are eligible
to be seen at the free clinic—to accept care provided at no charge? To suggest that there is a single "free clinic patient" profile or response is to over-
look the obvious: free clinic patients—like all patients—represent a wide
range of personal characteristics, personalities, and experiences. With the
exception of not having the resources to access private medical care, they
are no more of a single type than are the patients at any physician's office.

But the circumstance is different, and free clinic staff and volunteers who
were interviewed for this project talked about three patterns of patients'
emotional response to this circumstance: (1) some combination of frustration, resignation, and embarrassment; (2) a sense of entitlement and lack of
appreciation by a small number; and (3) heartfelt appreciation by many.

Frustration, Resignation, Embarrassment

Many free clinic patients, especially when they begin receiving care at the
clinic, convey an uncomfortableness about being there. This may stem from
frustration with the health care system or with their job or lack of a job, or
even with the amount of time they have to wait at the clinic before being
seen. Sometimes, the attitude is more of resignation to their inability to pay
for care or depression about having to be seen at the clinic. On rare occasions, the frustration or resignation is manifested in feelings of anger about
the way they have been treated by the private medical care system or the social services system, and sometimes this anger is vented on free clinic staff
and volunteers. Underlying these emotions often seems to be a feeling of
embarrassment of having to ask for something for free—embarrassment that
they have not acquired the financial wherewithal to be able to afford private
medical care.

> We have patients who come here and feel so humiliated that they explain them-
> selves through the entire evening, "I never come here." "This is the first time I
> have ever had to come here." "Normally, I have insurance or can pay my way."
> And, once in a while, we have angry patients who do not want to be here, but
> they express that in other ways. "Why is it taking so long?" "This is a long wait."
> "This is ridiculous." We usually end up finding out later that they are angry they
> have had to come here. (Maggie Caldarella, Clinical Coordinator, Bradley Free
> Clinic, Roanoke, Virginia)

> Though most of our patients are very grateful, some do express frustration with
> the system. They feel denigrated by the way that they have been treated as they
> go through the government bureaucracy, for example, being insulted in the
> process to get food stamps. They feel they are treated as something less than
> equal human beings. They are degraded. Are they embarrassed to come here?
> That depends on the patient. The nice building makes it easier to attend the

clinic. Some are embarrassed just initially; it is hardest for people who have never had to ask for anything. (Carla Bice, Executive Director, St. Joseph Health Center, South Bend, Indiana)

We use the model in which people register during certain hours, and whoever registers can be seen. We don't open our doors until 5:00 p.m., because once you let people in, they need to be seen, and we just don't have the staff to do that. So there is a period of time, a half an hour or more, depending on what time they get here, that they are standing on the street corner or on the street where their neighbors, their friends, their minister might pass by and see them. That can be a horrible thing for people to have to deal with. These people want to pay their own way. A lot of them don't feel comfortable out there being observed by the community. It hurts for them to come. They don't want to give up the idea that they can take care of themselves. (Jean Lee, Executive Director, Free Medical Clinic of Northern Shenandoah Valley, Winchester, Virginia)

When we see anger, it is typically anger at their situation rather than anger at any particular person. We do get the brunt of it once in a while when things don't get done quickly enough, for example. The majority of our patients are very embarrassed to be in this situation, especially those who are just now needing service. (Carol McHaley, DuPage Community Clinic, Wheaton, Illinois)

Some of our patients are embarrassed to have to contact us. I get many calls that go something like, "I can't believe that I am having to call you, but I am a single mom, and I simply don't have enough money to take my kids to the doctor." (Cam Buenzli, Healthnet of Janesville, Inc., Janesville, Wisconsin)

People like what they get here, but nobody likes having to come here. In the community at large, there may be some type of stigma attached to patients who have to come here. It means in some way in life, they have come up short. Whether they have any control of that is another matter. So here they are. It is not because they have all of these options and have chosen this place because it was the best place to get care, or because it is the most convenient for them, or any of those other things that those of us who are fortunate enough to have coverage take into consideration when we select a care provider. People end up here because they have to be here. The choices that they have are much more limited and carry much more complicated consequences if they choose wrong. So I have a lot of thankful people, and I have a lot of people who would be even more thankful if they never had to come back.

All of the time, people vent about problems in trying to get care in the private sector. People have been referred here by someone else in the health care system, they have been bounced here, and nobody feels good about that. The difficulty is complicated by the fact that they also might not find what they need here. A guy goes to the emergency room with chest pains and walks out with prescriptions. He asks how he can get them filled, and the response is to call the free clinic. We have a pharmacy here, but it is for our patients. So somebody will walk through the door with a handful of prescriptions that may very well be the difference between healthy living and living or not, and there is not anything for them here either. It is tough when all we can offer is a sympathetic ear. (Marty Hiller, Executive Director, Free Clinic of Greater Cleveland, Cleveland, Ohio)

Free clinics are sensitive to the emotions of their patients and consciously work to overcome any feelings of embarrassment that their patients feel. Their strategies include open discussion about patients' feelings, emphasizing to all staff and volunteers the importance of treating patients with respect and dignity, and providing top-notch medical care in as comfortable a surrounding as possible.

It is very important that we respect where they are, and we treat them with respect because they are our fellow human beings and our neighbors. By the grace of God go any of us. Any of us could lose our access to health care. We work hard to make them comfortable and to say that this is an okay place for now, that they need to be here, and that we are here to help them wherever life has them at the moment. We all have bad days. Not every free clinic patient is always perfectly polite. Then again, not every person with many fewer woes in life is always perfectly polite. (Lee Elmore, Executive Director, North Coast Health Ministry, Lakewood, Ohio)

People can tell if you care or if you don't. It makes a difference when people know that you care, that you are doing what you can. Our patients respond to that because in many cases people have never really expressed care for them. They have been labeled, and they have been stereotyped. They are so used to the system turning its back on them. Some of them are very angry, and it takes awhile to establish rapport. (Judy Dillow, Director of the Medical Clinic, First Baptist Church of North Charleston Medical Clinic, North Charleston, South Carolina)

Some of the friends and neighbors who come to us come down and dejected. Some have little sense of self-worth and only a marginal amount of dignity. Then [after being seen at the clinic], they not only have dignity and a sense of self-worth, they tell us that. And they have a sense of purpose in their lives that they didn't have. They have a place that they can come to and someone who will listen to them. One person said it was the first time that people had treated her like she was really somebody instead of just being a number on a chart. There is a lot behind the quiet demeanor, and all you have to do is ask and be kind and they will share it with you. (Jack McConnell, Founder, Volunteers in Medicine Clinic, Hilton Head Island, South Carolina)

Do the patients express anger at the existing health care system—no. Do they feel embarrassment to have to come to the free clinic—softly stated, yes. Are they appreciative—yes, but they are not servile about it. They don't tug at their forelocks and bow as we walk by. Nor would we wish that. There is a degree of dignity in that you are treated by doctors and nurses, who work and then choose to come in to the clinic. Now that we are in a treatment center second to none, that conveys dignity. (John Garvin, MD, former medical director, Bradley Free Clinic, Roanoke, Virginia)

A Sense of Entitlement and Lack of Appreciation

Although it is not common, many free clinics occasionally do encounter patients who convey a sense of entitlement to clinic services and a lack of appreciation for them. Typically, these patients perceive that the free clinic has a responsibility or obligation to provide medical care for them and to do so in a way that maximizes patient convenience. Although only a very small percentage of patients seem to feel this sense of entitlement, they are the patients most likely to complain about services and to be discourteous to staff members and volunteers.

Free clinic directors are protective of their staff and volunteers and usually deal straightforwardly with patients who express rudeness toward them. Often, all it takes is an explanation about the voluntary basis of the free clinic— that most of the medical providers and others working at the clinic are there providing a service without compensation and that the clinic is not a government-sponsored program providing care to which anyone is entitled.

A handful of our patients do think it is an entitlement. "I'm here, you serve me to the best of your ability," and they are not grateful or appreciative at all. A few don't want to sit near other patients—they don't want to catch anything. It seems to be a way of thinking that they are a little bit better than others. Those with an entitlement attitude routinely think this is a government program and do not understand the nature of the clinic. I explain the clinic to them, and I also say to them that in my own private doctor's office, I wait an hour in the waiting room, and forty-five minutes in the exam room, and then there is a copay and the drugs are not free. (Maggie Caldarella, Clinical Coordinator, Bradley Free Clinic, Roanoke, Virginia)

There is often an initial level of mistrust that they will be provided with quality medical care, with substandard doctors. They almost expect second-class care. Some do not really understand that the free clinic is not a government program. These patients sometimes get frustrated if they can't get everything they need. (Barb Tylenda, Health Care Network, Inc., Racine, Wisconsin)

The vast majority of our patients are quite pleased and happy with the clinic. Some are surprised that it is a nice environment, that they don't have to wait in line. They make an appointment, and hopefully they are seen within fifteen to twenty minutes. They get all services for free. A small minority are not happy. They are upset by waiting ten minutes before being seen. Often, they have the misunderstanding that the clinic is government funded. "You have to see me, you get government money." The entitlement attitude is often linked to this mis-perception. (James Beckner, Executive Director, Fan Free Clinic, Richmond, Virginia)

Ninety-nine percent of our patients are grateful for services they get. They do a comment card, rate the services they have received, and make comments. They are very grateful and do not feel we are belittling them. A few—many second- and third-generation welfare recipients—have an entitlement attitude. They have grown up with the attitude that everybody owes them something. They are used to pitching a fit to get what they want. What they learn is that gets you less attention than those who wait their turn. We will discontinue services for pa-tients who come in and get in the face of our volunteers or be threatening or disrespectful. Our volunteers do not have to be here. I don't have any problem saying to a patient that disrespectful behavior is unacceptable here. (Sandy Mot-ley, Executive Director, Davidson Medical Ministries Clinic, Inc., Lexington, North Carolina)

Most of our patients are very appreciative. Recently, one couple came in with six prescriptions, got five of them filled, complained that they could not get the sixth one filled, and walked out without saying thank you. This shows the im-portance of educating our patients about who we are. All of the people here give enormously of themselves to make the clinic possible. Some patients have said to us that they are sad about the way that the few ungrateful or abusive pa-tients treat the staff, and they appreciate that we don't simply take it. (Jean Lee, Executive Director, Free Medical Clinic of Northern Shenandoah Valley, Win-chester, Virginia)

Appreciation

The overwhelming percentage of free clinic patients are very appreciative of the medical care they receive in the free clinic and of the caring manner of the staff and volunteers. Sometimes, they articulate their feelings in detail, sometimes it is just in the genuineness of their thank-you, sometimes it is in special gestures they make. Several free clinic directors have experienced sit-uations in which patients wept because they were so overcome that the clinic staff and volunteers were really going to help them.

A lady came in to us with abdominal pain. She worked part-time at K-Mart, so she did not have enough hours to get insurance there. We examined her, did x-rays, and determined that she had gallstones. For the rest of us, if we were di-agnosed with gallstones, we might say let's take out the gallbladder, who needs it anyway. But we called the surgeon, and he suggested some medication to try to deal with the gallstones. It was very expensive, and there was no way that she could afford it. As luck would have it, there was an indigent medication pro-gram for that medication. We got it for her. Then, she developed some other conditions that became life-threatening. Ultimately, she got a medical card [which enabled her to receive private care] and no longer qualified for the clinic. She called us on a monthly basis, until she died, and reported on how she was doing, how she appreciated the fact that we had seen her when she didn't have insurance. We had helped to get her diagnosed and to get her into treatment as soon as it was discovered. When this lady passed away, what was left of her estate was $237. Her sister brought that money here and said that her sister had always said that if anything ever happened to her, if there was anything left in her estate, she wanted the clinic to have it.

Our patients are just like any other patients; they are a smorgasbord; every patient is an individual. Some patients are angry—mostly that they are having to use free care. They are hurt. Others have multiple illnesses and mental health problems and are struggling to get through each day. They are very appreciative of the clinic and of our very special staff. Many say, "I can't believe that people cared enough to do this for us." (Sheri Wood, Executive Director, Kansas City Free Health Clinic, Kansas City, Missouri)

We had a male patient who was just a little bit over qualifying for services here. He had a bad lung condition, and we went ahead and treated him. Eventually, he got disability payments, and when he received his settlement, he came in and said he just wanted to tell us good-bye and get his records, and said, "While I am here, you have been so good to me that I want to give you a little something." Well, our administrative assistant took the money but didn't pay any attention to how much it was. After he left, we counted it, and it was $300. Now, just the last time we had seen him, he had needed medication that we did not have here. They had kerosene heat in their house, but they opted not to buy kerosene, so they could buy his medicine that week. They did without heat, and when he got that settlement, he gave us $300. That was a fortune to them.

Most of our patients are so thankful that we are here for them on that particular day or that particular moment in their life and for the long-lasting contact that we have with them. You can really see how just one contact with someone for a short amount of time can mean so much. (Leigh Ann Surgent, St. Anthony Free Clinic, San Francisco, California)

Most patients are very grateful. People come in who have lost their job and are having to come to grips with the fact that they cannot make it on their own. Sometimes multiple overwhelming things are happening. One lady said, "If I didn't have the free clinic, I don't know what I would do." She received a $500 tax refund and gave it all to the clinic. (Jeri White, Executive Director, The Community Clinic of High Point, High Point, North Carolina)

Our patients are fantastic people. Sometimes volunteers come to us thinking they will find an entitled, surly population who expect to be taken care of. The uninsured are totally different. They are falling between the cracks. They come in and are so incredibly appreciative for what you are doing for them. The doctors are always saying that they don't get this many thank-yous in their own private offices. And, they pay back by being compliant. They cannot pay in money, but they can take their medications, they can stop smoking, they can lose weight, whatever we ask them to do. That is not to say that they are all the same, but more often than not, that is the case. So, they are just warm, wonderful people to work with. (Karen Gottlieb, Americares Free Clinics, New Canaan, Connecticut)

One Christmas a mother brought in her little four-year-old son. We were just closing the morning clinic. I said, "Good morning. How are you? Haven't I taken care of you?" She said that we had, and I responded that I thought I had seen this handsome young man before. I asked if she was here for herself, and she said, "No, it is for him." I asked what was the problem. She said that he doesn't have a problem, he has something for you. He reached in his pocket and pulled out four crumpled one-dollar bills. I said, "Oh my goodness, what is this?" She said, "I gave him the four dollars so we could go to Wal-Mart, and he could pick out something he wanted for Christmas. He said he wanted to take it and give it to my doctor."

MEASURING OUTCOMES

The obvious thrust of free clinics is to improve patient health: to diagnose accurately, to help determine the proper course of treatment, and to provide the identified treatment or help to obtain it elsewhere in the medical community. It is very important to free clinics that services be provided in a respectful manner so that patients feel comfortable coming to the clinic and so that they develop positive relationships with clinic staff and volunteers. A logical hope is that individuals and families who are unable to access the private care system do not feel the burden of having unmet medical needs and the knowledge that they can do nothing about it. Beyond these obvious goals, many free clinics intend to impact patients in at least two other ways: helping patients to stay in or return to the labor force and enhancing the sense of personal empowerment by helping patients to make health-promoting changes in their lifestyle.

Labor Force Participation

Sensitivity to the working poor—to individuals who work full-time or part-time for a low wage and without health benefits—is the hallmark of most free clinics. It is their understanding that many people lack financial resources and lack health insurance not because they are unwilling to work for a living but because the jobs for which they are qualified are not valued with high compensation and do not offer an insurance benefit. In some cases, even when there is employer-provided health insurance, many low-income individuals and families risk everything by not securing it because the employee portion is too costly. For many families the thousands of dollars per year that the employee portion costs competes with the purchase of food, shelter, basic utilities, clothing, and other needs. Many wage workers cannot take time off work to see a medical provider without a wage deduction for the hours missed. Then, the lack of needed care causes illnesses to worsen and sometimes prevents workers from staying in the labor force at all. Free clinics try to marshal needed resources so that these individuals and their families can derive the personal benefits of employment and continue to make a contribution to society. Some of the patient stories most fondly remembered by clinic staff and volunteers are those in which care received at the free clinic enabled a patient to stay in or return to the labor force.

A young woman used to come to the clinic in the early years after the college group passed. She was older, she wasn't a teen, she was in her early twenties, and she would work day jobs to go out and earn money. On one very hot day, she came in, and she was wearing long sleeves. Another volunteer and I were working, and she said, "Oh, it is so hot out," and I asked if she needed a short-sleeve blouse. She said that she did not, that she didn't wear anything short-sleeve. We asked why, and she rolled up her sleeve and showed us where she had cheloid tissue all over her arms due to attempts at suicide. We had never seen anything like it. The other volunteer told her about a philanthropist whom she had read about who was connected with a local university, paying doctors to help people who needed some type of plastic surgery. She remembered the name, made the telephone call, followed through, and made the appointment for this young woman. It ended up that there was nothing that could be done, there were just too many suicide and track marks from drugs. The young lady told us that it was the first time in her life that anybody had ever gone out of their way to do something for her. Then she told us the story of her life which wasn't very pleasant. We did get her into some counseling. Later, she came back and told us what we had done turned her life around—that she saw that there was something good and that we had helped her tremendously. She was able to get a job and get to a point where her arms did not bother her that much. She uncovered them.

A woman whose lungs were in terrible condition came in to us. She had asthma, she was a smoker, and I said to her that she needed to quit smoking—that it was not good for her children, and it prevented her from getting better and going back to work. I told her about our vocational rehabilitation center that would help get her back into the labor force. She wrote down all of the information. She came back several months later. Her lungs were cleared up. She left here the last time and started to light up but did not. She said, "You know you are right, the only person who can take care of this is me." She said, "I decided to quit smoking, I won't allow anyone to smoke now in my house. I lost some of my friends, but I realized it is important for my kids not to have anyone smoking around here. I went to vocational rehabilitation. I got a job, and I now have insurance."

A lady who cleans offices every evening came to the clinic during her work time. She sat in the waiting room and tapped her feet because she was anxious to get back to her job. She did not want to get in trouble for missing work to go to clinic. She had diabetes and hypertension. Whenever she came in, she always had a lot of swelling in her legs. She also had very arthritic knees. She was determined that these things were not going to stand between her and cleaning those offices because that was her paycheck. She is a very strong-willed woman. She has definite ideas of what was causing her ailments—how the purple pill was not going to work as well as the pink pill. She is always a challenge and always a pleasure.

We often get patients who have not been able to work because of diabetes. They enter our program. They get stabilized. They get the help they need, and then they go out and get a job and eventually get benefits. They leave the clinic and can get private care. We had one man who was a patient here for two years. When he initially came in, his diabetes was out of control, and he had kidney damage. He had been working part-time because he was not able to keep a full-time job. When he left us, he got a full-time job with health benefits and went to a doctor as a paying patient.

We had a client who had been a patient for several years. She is in her fifties, is diabetic, and she works most of the time in a laundry in a local nursing home. She has worked there for twelve years. She does not have health insurance, that is not an option with her job. We have treated her in our general clinic for four years. She would get her blood sugar checked twice per month; she would get her medicine and go home. She was one of the first clients moved to our chronic disease clinic. Last summer, in August, she came in with an ingrown toenail which should not have been a big deal. But, because her diabetes was not very well controlled at that time, the toe became grossly infected. We had her out of work for three months on short-term disability. Because of her job, she was not drawing any kind of disability benefits. We did help her with expenses. She came to the clinic every week for three months. We gave her antibiotics. When it was not adequately responding, we sent her for free to an orthopedist—one of our referral physicians—who treated her, continued to see her, and treated her again. The toe healed, and she went to back to work. Without us, she would likely have lost her toe and maybe her foot. She could never have paid the orthopedist to have that done. She would have been in the hospital on IV antibiotics. Because of us, she was able to be treated, to get well, to go back to work, and now to control her diabetes.

We saw a patient in our clinic who had asthma. She had been going to the emergency room almost every week. She would go, and they would nebulize her and do whatever they needed to do to stop her wheezing. They would write a prescription for inhalers and send her on her way. She would go back the next week and go back the next week. Finally, one of the nurses asked why she was there again, that she was just in last week. She told them that it was because they had given her a prescription, and she didn't have the money to purchase the inhaler. So the nurse said that she should come to the free clinic and get her nebulizer here. She came to us. She was a fairly serious asthmatic who had had trouble holding a job because of her illness. So we gave her the medicine, scheduled her for our continuity clinic where she would see the same doctor to get her asthma under control. She came in one day and said, "I have a job." Everybody congratulated her and thought that was just wonderful. She came back three months later and said that she now had insurance and would not be able to come to the clinic anymore. The free clinic helps to break the cycle of illness, to keep people well, to keep them working, to get insured. These patients need a place where they can get their medication and get well.

Patient Empowerment

Many patients who come to free clinics do not have strong feelings of empowerment with their lives in general and with their medical care in particular. Most have experienced occasions when they simply could not afford to obtain needed medical care. Many have accumulated bills with physicians or hospitals or other providers and lack the means to pay the bill. Many have gone to hospital emergency rooms for primary care because that was the only care available. Little about life is easy, and the idea of really being in charge of one's life is very difficult. Staff and volunteers at free clinics are aware that seeking care there may in some ways add to the feelings of disempowerment.

But part of the mission for many free clinics is to empower their patients. They recognize the important life benefits and health benefits of patients taking greater charge of their health: by becoming more knowledgeable about health and illness, by becoming more assertive when conversing with medical providers, and by trying to live a healthier lifestyle. Clinics want their patients to understand that most diseases from which people suffer are related to lifestyle: the foods we eat, the amount of alcohol we drink, the tobacco and other drugs that we use, the amount of exercise that we get, and so on. Many clinics have a paid or volunteer health educator—sometimes a nurse or nurse practitioner will provide patient education—and some clinics, such as the Kalamazoo [Michigan] Free Clinic, have established behavioral health programs. Several clinics have staff or volunteer dieticians to work with patients.

St. Joseph Health Center in South Bend, Indiana, has constructed an exercise room for its patients. It includes three treadmills, several exercise bicycles, a stairstepper, and a rowing machine, and it is overseen by a cardiac rehabilitation nurse. A diabetic educator and a dietician also work with the patients. The clinic also provides space for meetings of other groups such as Alcoholics Anonymous, support groups for families of alcoholics, AIDS testing and counseling, literacy counseling and reading programs, English as a Second Language programs, mental health counseling, women's support groups, and smoking cessation individual and group counseling programs.

West Virginia Health Right in Charleston, West Virginia, offers several different classes for patients such as tobacco cessation, Weight Watchers, monitoring diabetes, and physical exercise. Patients are told they must consider their health-related lifestyle and to make some healthy change no matter how small it is.

The Hollywood Sunset Free Clinic in Los Angeles provides garden plots for patients with no other space to grow their own vegetables. It also for many years has sponsored a health education theater group.

> We have found that education in an entertaining fashion really draws their attention. Our low-income patients do not have money to go out for entertainment. Many have anywhere from three to five kids, so we provide that form of education and entertainment for them. We write all of our own skits, and we cover a whole range of issues—being HIV-positive, child abuse, being gay or lesbian. Each issue is covered in a small skit no longer than fifteen minutes. After each one, we have a period where the actors ask the audience for participation, staying still in their role, and so the audience, for example, may ask questions about child abuse to the actor who was portraying a child abuser. It is very effective. We have been doing it for many years both in Spanish and English. (Tacy Padua, Executive Director, Hollywood Sunset Free Clinic, Los Angeles, California)

Despite the importance of lifestyle, research has shown that many physicians continue to focus on symptoms and organs and do not have in-depth discussions with patients about their health-harming behaviors. One might think that it would be even more difficult for staff and volunteers in free clinics to have these conversations and to do meaningful patient education. In some cases, the number of patients to be seen relative to the number of providers does make this extremely difficult if not impossible. However, many free clinics have designed specialty clinics or special health education programs or other strategies to inform patients about the importance of lifestyle and to assist them in making changes.

> We are not here just to patch people up but to help people take care of themselves and to make sure they get to appropriate resources in the community. An important part of our job is to educate people to take care of themselves. (Karon Jones, Clinical Services Director, Free Clinic of Franklin County, North Carolina)

> Many of the patients who come into our clinic really just need basic education in how to care for themselves in a healthy way. It is really hard in the inner city. The stress is incredible, most of the parents are working two jobs, and they live in crowded conditions. So there is a need for an outlet and a way to learn how to eat healthy and to exercise and to work stress out so that is not a negative thing. (Tacy Padua, Executive Director, Hollywood Sunset Free Clinic, Los Angeles, California)

Our focus here is on empowering people, putting medicine into lay terms, hopefully making them more effective patients in other settings. Our services are very client-oriented. We put the client first, their needs first, we try to make sure that all of their needs are met, and it is a really gratifying experience as a provider working at a peer level. People come out of appointments with a much better feeling about themselves; they come out happier knowing that someone cares; they have a better sense of what is going on in themselves; and they feel less scared, less frustrated. (Sairah Husain, Director of the Information and Referral Collective, Berkeley Free Clinic, Berkeley, California)

The biggest reason for the high rate of diabetes among our patients is lifestyle. Many have always lived a lifestyle that is very high in carbohydrates, lots of beans, lots of potatoes, lots of bread, which converts to sugar. Some of them live a very sedentary lifestyle. A lot of it is lack of education. We estimate that about 33 percent of our patients are functionally illiterate. So handing them a brochure that says you have type 2 diabetes and this is what you do for it, I may as well put it in the trash can because it is not going to do any good, they are not going to read it and, if they read it, they would not understand it. So education is a big piece of it. They don't know. If someone says they have diabetes, all they know is that they are not to eat sweets. They don't know that going to dinner and having pintos and potatoes and cornbread, they just ate three starches, and every bit of that is going to convert to sugar. They may not have pie, but they may as well have. And they don't eat a lot of protein. So they don't know how to eat. Plus, eating a healthy diet is more expensive than eating what you can get your hands on. It may be a young mother who is struggling, trying to make ends meet and support a family. She is going to put three pot pies in the oven, which she can get three for a dollar at Food Lion, instead of buying chicken and baking it and making a green salad, which is going to cost her much more.

We have done surveys of our clients as to what they eat. Especially among our seniors, we find people who sometimes eat cat food because it is cheap, or people eating one meal a day. I think the fact that diabetes and hypertension are as rampant as they are is a combination of not being able to financially afford a balanced diet and not having the education to understand what they need to do to manage it.

We have a chronic disease clinic with a pharmacy director who is just a phenomenal person. She is a certified diabetic educator. She goes through the diet with our patients. She literally helps them to go to the grocery store, and she talks about what is a good choice and what is not a good choice and how to do serving sizes. She helps them to understand what they are eating and helps them to figure out how to arrange that to balance their diet. We are seeing phenomenal results in our clinic with a steady progression in reducing their sugars. They are getting their medicines, and they are getting routine follow-up. (Sandy Motley, Executive Director, Davidson Medical Ministries, Lexington, North Carolina)

One woman walked into our clinic with a walker, and both of her knees had advanced degenerative disease. She weighed 250 pounds and was not helping herself. She was in her fifties, an attractive woman, just heavy, and now crippled and in a lot of pain. She came to the orthopedic clinic, and she started asking the doctor what she could do with her knees. The doctor told her that her knees needed to be replaced, that there was no question about it. She asked if we would pay for that. He told her that he didn't know but that he could do the surgery for her but wouldn't. She asked what kind of answer that was. He told her that there was a lot of risk involved in the surgery and that she needed to make a commitment to helping herself. She asked if the clinic would pay if she made that commitment. He told her that if she made the commitment that he would guarantee that he would do the surgery. So she asked what the commitment was. He told her that she needed to lose 100 pounds and the reason was because when he did the surgery, he would be replacing both knees, and about four hours after the surgery, she would need to get out of bed and to walk in order to avoid problems, to avoid complications, and to avoid clots. He said, "I am taking a tremendous risk to do this surgery for you, and you will be my patient for the rest of your life. If anything goes wrong, you are going to come get me. So you must lose 100 pounds." She angrily said, "Well, how am I going to lose 100 pounds?" He told her she needed to watch what she ate, she needed to exercise, and she needed to come to the clinic for our Weight Watchers program and that we would help her with all of this. Six months later, she had lost 107 pounds. She had both of her knees replaced. She is now a completely different person with a whole different life, and she is doing very well.

A woman came to us feeling tired, fatigued. We ran some routine blood tests to try to figure out why she was feeling so tired. She was a working mother with two kids of her own, and she was raising two of another relative's kids. Her husband had died suddenly four years ago, and she still was grieving about that. When her lab tests came back, she was diabetic. Our physician got her back in, talked with her personally, and got her into our diabetic clinic. She came back with concerns about vision. The clinic got her an ophthalmology exam, and everything was fine. She still was concerned about the diabetes diagnosis. We worked closely with her. Two months later, she was doing great. She made dietary changes. Her lab numbers all looked good. She was able to keep working. We were able to take away the financial barrier of receiving services.

I think the main thing about the clinic is that we are taking people who are near poverty and who are trying to go to work and do their job, but they have an illness or have a problem that if untreated might keep them from work. Our role is simply to do what we can to help. For instance, you have a forty-year-old who has type 2 diabetes. For most of our patients, that would put them immediately into poverty and on welfare because they can't afford their medications. They lose their job and they are left with deciding if they put shoes on their kids or buy them a backpack for school or buy their medications. Our role is simply to be there and to say, "Look, it is not going to cost you a dime. All you have to do is have the motivation. We're going to explain and give you the education to know why it is important." For our average patient with high blood pressure plus type 2 diabetes, the cost of the medications alone is somewhere in the neighborhood of $3,500 a year. The cost of seeing a doctor just to keep up with the conditions is in the neighborhood of $1,000+ per year for a total of $4,500 for someone to pay without insurance out of pocket and that does not include any acute illness care. If the person is making $21,000 a year, nowadays you can't put food on the table and have a house over your head and take care of two or three kids and pay $4,500 a year in medical costs. So they do exactly what all of us would do in that situation: they don't take certain medications, they just neglect it as long as they are relatively healthy and until they lose the feeling in their feet or start going blind. The large majority of our patients when they were given the diagnosis of diabetes simply expected to wait until they were disabled and to collect disability. That was the game plan. We work with them to show that diabetes can be controlled.

9

The Future Path
of Free Health Clinics

> How can one little clinic make a difference? Well, it makes a huge difference to each community that starts a free clinic.
>
> (Kevin Kelleher, MD, Bradley Free Clinic)

The future course for America's free health clinics will be shaped by a complex interplay of factors at both the societal and organizational levels. How these factors play out will have a significant impact on the stability and possible expansion of free health clinics and on the particular role that they play within the health care system. Four of these factors seem most important: (1) health care access policy decisions made at the federal and state levels, (2) demographic changes within the United States population, (3) the maintenance and possible expansion of corporate, foundation, and public financial support for free clinics, and (4) the level of development of free clinic associations and supporting organizations. These factors interrelate but, taken together, should represent significant influences on the future role of free health clinics in the health care system.

HEALTH CARE ACCESS POLICY

Federal Policy

As described in chapter 3, countries around the world offer a wide variety of approaches for structuring and focusing their health care systems. Some countries, like Great Britain and Germany, have health care systems in which health care planning and health care resources are largely under government control, although there is a small private sector. Some countries, like Canada and Japan, have health care systems that are essentially private in nature, although there is significant direction given by the government. However, all of these countries have in common that they identify health care as being a right of all citizens rather than a privilege for those with sufficient financial resources. Among modern countries, only the United States fails to make this commitment to its people, and there is little reason to foresee that changing. Congress seems unable and unwilling to formulate broad-scale changes in the nation's health care system, and it is increasingly clear that America's middle class and upper class are not willing to pay more or be inconvenienced so that all persons have access to private care.

This is not meant to suggest that health care systems in other countries do not have problems. Almost all countries are struggling currently with high health care costs and with having sufficient health care resources to prevent long waits for treatment. But no country emphasizes profit making in the health care system like the United States, no country has millions of people (or any number of people) who cannot access needed health care because they do not have adequate financial resources, and no country has depended on volunteer-driven, community-based agencies like free health clinics to try to get essential preventive and curative care to the medically indigent. This is a profound difference in structure and a profound difference in values, and it leads to profound differences in access to health care for millions of people.

Since 1932, there have been unceasing efforts made by individuals in Congress to introduce and gain passage of a universal coverage health care bill. On a few occasions—most recently in the early years of the Clinton Administration—there appeared to be sufficient support in the nation and in Congress that legislation might be passed. But such legislation has never received ultimate passage, and typically the period of renewed interest is followed by a period when universal coverage moves to the back burner. For the most part, staff and volunteers in free health clinics—people who tend to watch health care policy very closely—hold little hope or anticipation that the United States will join the world's other countries in guaranteeing health care to all.

> From all of my twenty-five years in health care, I can say that obviously the health care system in this country is broken. I think we all know that. It is probably going to take more political will than anyone has in the foreseeable future to change that because it is so tied in with capitalism . . . and what we have defaulted to is an unspoken system of rationing with those not having the necessary financial resources—money or insurance—not being able to get care. (Glenn Pierce, Executive Director, Asheville-Buncombe Community Christian Ministries Free Clinic, Asheville, North Carolina)

I see the free clinic movement arising out of a society in the 1960s that was more embracing of the welfare of all. Unfortunately, I don't feel that captures the attitude of our current society. I see people as having become more and more self-absorbed, and more focused on the individual, and as long as they are successful and make money, that is where the focus is. I feel there will always be pockets of individuals who are relatively more progressive than that and care about the well-being of all, but I don't see that as a really strong ongoing societal movement. (Diana Amodia, MD, Haight-Ashbury Free Clinics, Inc., San Francisco, California)

There is just not now a political agenda to solve the problem of the working poor. There is not the political will, and there is not sufficient will from the people to do that. (Kevin Kelleher, MD, Medical Director, Bradley Free Clinic, Roanoke, Virginia)

We are a very affluent country with a horrible health care system. Dental care is really lacking. We have so much money in our country, yet we don't provide basic health care services. We see people in our clinic who, if they had to pay for their prescriptions, they would start taking their pills every other day, because that is what they would have to do to pay the rent, buy food, and clothe the kids. It just doesn't seem that anyone ought to have to make that kind of choice. But we don't change the system. (Becky Weybright, Executive Director, Charlottesville Free Clinic, Charlottesville, Virginia)

Many free clinics were created with the idea that they would phase out should universal coverage ever become a reality. They self-envisioned being only a temporary agency that would try to meet the needs until a more comprehensive system was put into place. Some still see it that way, but most have come to believe that, even in the very unlikely case that a universal coverage bill would be enacted, that there would likely be so many qualifications, limitations, and exclusions that many people would still be unable to access basic health care. Whether it is exclusion of some services—such as mental health care, adult dentistry, medications, or patient education—or not having adequate facilities and resources for some groups of people— such as the homeless, undocumented immigrants, non-English speakers, or people with substance abuse problems—there is a perception that there will be a sizable niche that free clinics will be called upon to serve. Most would concur with the words of James Beckner, executive director of the Fan Free Clinic in Richmond, Virginia:

Having insurance does not guarantee equal access to health care. Insurance does not mean attitudinal access to health care. Insurance does not mean having adequate resources that are available. There are still barriers. Nothing would make me happier than to close this place down because it is not needed. I would love to go out of business. Realistically, I don't think it will happen.

The bills that Congress passes are usually so full of holes, and what the politicians forget to write in is ably made up for by the ineptness of the people who implement those bills. I rather expect that there will always be a need for free clinics. It is due to my abiding disdain for much of what the federal and state governments try to get done. They are constantly out of money, every time we turn around, taxes are going up, and they spend money on projects that just seem totally pointless. I can't help but think that the ineptitude will always be with us. (John M. "Lucky" Garvin, MD, former medical director and Board President, Bradley Free Clinic, Roanoke, Virginia)

Even if a national health bill is passed, there will always be people who fall through the cracks. One of the goals of free clinics is to work ourselves out of business. If there was legislation, the face of free clinics might change, but there will always be people who fall through the cracks. (Sandy Motley, Executive Director, Davidson Medical Ministries Clinic, Inc., Lexington, North Carolina)

People will always fall through the cracks. Right now, California has a program so that women of reproductive age can get reimbursed for certain gynecological services. But women who are not of reproductive age or who have had a hysterectomy cannot get Pap smears through this program. We have a large number of women who fall within that group. Like all free clinics, we believe that if there is a need, we have to try and meet it. (Tacy Padua, Executive Director, Hollywood Sunset Free Clinic, Los Angeles, California)

If a national health insurance bill was passed, it is hard to speculate on what the bill would be like. But I think there will always be people who are not part of the system. I can't imagine our country changing so radically that that would not be the case. Perhaps it would be people who live on the streets or those abusing drugs. (Pastor Keith Goretzka, First Baptist Church of North Charleston Medical Clinic, North Charleston, South Carolina)

Should Congress pass some form of national health insurance, I think there will always be folks who drop out of the system. I think free clinics would change, though I am not sure how exactly they would look. Right now, if I am doing 25,000 patient visits annually, where would they all go? People with HIV, with substance abuse problems, with mental health problems don't always fall within the health care system. Physicians' offices do not always have all of the components. (Sheri Wood, Executive Director, Kansas City Free Health Clinic, Kansas City, Missouri)

If a national health insurance bill would pass, would there be a need for free clinics? It depends on the definition of who qualifies, because we always have people who fall through the cracks. Our clinic is close to a border of another country. People come no matter what, they need to come, they have no other means of economics. Right now, there is a war in Honduras. There is terrible hunger, people are dying of hunger every day, children are dying every day. They are going to come here because we are still the land of milk and honey for many, and Los Angeles has the opportunity for work. . . . There is also the group of working-class people who work but do not receive any health insurance. Where can they go? We are now the biggest area of the country for garment workers, surpassing even New York. They are not organized in any form of union, and they do not get any medical care insurance whatsoever. They work twelve hours a day in all kinds of terrible conditions, dusty, feathers if they are doing comforters, whatever. They have to see somebody. (Virginia Halstead, Administrative Assistant, Hollywood Sunset Free Clinic, Los Angeles, California)

If we passed a national health insurance bill, I don't think they would tear down all of the free clinics around the country. I would hope that what would happen is that we would be integrated into the whole health care system. . . . I think that community efforts like this are so much more cost-efficient, though it is hard to get the money that we need, and there seems to be much more of a passion for patients in places like this. (Parker Sparrow, Executive Director, The Free Medical Clinic, Columbia, South Carolina)

State Policy

Given the small likelihood of national legislation to guarantee health care access, many state governments have become more active agents in health care reform. State legislatures have some advantages and some disadvantages in trying to secure access to health care for their people. Obviously, states have less access than the federal government to a huge pool of funds, and wealth and income vary enormously from state to state. States can plan programs only within their borders, so that the large number of people who permanently or temporarily cross state borders creates complex coverage and eligibility questions. For programs such as the purchase of prescription medicines from another country, it is much more difficult for each state to enter into an agreement than it would be for the federal government to develop a single policy or formulate an agreement. In periods of economic downturn, state budgets can be especially hard hit, and discretionary funds for social and health programming can be very tight or nonexistent. When certain progressive states do develop creative programs, the benefits typically are not experienced by residents of other states.

However, legislative change at the state level does not have to contend with the large federal bureaucracy and sometimes not with the games of power and word spinning that dominate the national scene. In a sense they are closer to the particular needs of state residents and theoretically should be able to tailor programs to specific needs. But, even at the state level, the willingness and ability of state politicians to acknowledge and address serious social programs vary tremendously, and an insufficiency of available funds has frequently thwarted even conscientious efforts to enable all residents to obtain health care.

In the coming years, action at the state level may impact free clinics in at least four important ways: (1) enactment of health care access legislation, (2) programs to secure pharmaceuticals at lower cost, (3) changes in Medicaid eligibility rules or extent of coverage, and (4) direct efforts to increase access to health care services by channeling funds through free clinics.

State Health Policy Legislation

Frustrated by the lack of federal action, several states have developed their own programs to increase the number of people able to access private care. Since 1974, Hawaii has required most employers to provide their employees with health care benefits. Combining these with Medicare and Medicaid, most Hawaiians have basic health care coverage. In more recent years, Tennessee, Washington, Massachusetts, Vermont, Minnesota, and other states have attempted to open access to health care for more people. While implementation and sustainability of these programs is often threatened by funding shortages, the effort does reflect an interest in addressing the problem. About one-quarter of the states had passed programs to increase access to health care for poor children before Congress set up the State Children's Health Insurance Program. Maine is in the process of creating several health care reforms with the aim of having universal coverage within the state within the next few years (Riley and Kilbreth 2004). Should both the will and funds exist, state legislation could reduce the number of people needing free clinic services.

State Purchase of Pharmaceuticals

Some states have already created or are in the process of creating programs to secure pharmaceuticals at lower cost or to enable more people to purchase medications using the traditional discount (about 20–25 percent off retail) required for Medicaid patients. Some states are attempting to steer Medicaid patients toward less expensive drugs that have proven to be effective. Some states and cities are making arrangements to purchase drugs from Canada (where cost controls lead to much less expensive drugs). The pharmaceutical industry has challenged efforts of these types in courts, and though states have usually prevailed in the end, it has been only after significant cost and delay. Many of the states have expressed disappointment with a lack of support from Washington and with what they consider to be unnecessary delays. Clearly, more effective federal-state communication on these innovative ideas could make medications more available at lower cost to those now unable to afford them. That could reduce the need for free clinic drug assistance.

Changes in Medicaid

Reduced state costs in the purchase of pharmaceuticals might relieve some of the pressure on state budgets created by Medicaid. If successful, this could lead states to reduce efforts to tighten eligibility standards for Medicaid, to constrict covered services, and to reduce payments to providers. Should that happen, more people may be able to secure needed services through Medicaid and not have to rely on free clinic services and pharmacies. But there is no guarantee that savings in Medicaid drug purchases will be reinvested in the Medicaid program. States may choose to spend the funds on education, homeland security, tax cuts, or other areas. Many analysts believe that, despite the potential savings in drug purchases, Medicaid eligibility will continue to tighten and that fewer low-income persons—rather than more—will be able to obtain needed care covered by Medicaid.

Direct Support for Free Clinics

Many people in state government are looking for the most cost-efficient means for trying to ensure access to health care for all persons. An option to help to accomplish this objective is the direct channeling of funds from state governments to free clinics. Some see this as a win-win position. The financial support would enable more free clinics to open and assist existing free clinics to expand their services. More people would be able to receive needed medical care. Because most free clinics are volunteer-dependent, they provide enormous "bang for the buck"—often four, five, six, or seven times in services the amount of money invested. No other existing option provides the same cost-benefit value. Direct channeling of funds to a state free clinic association for allocation to individual free clinics, as is currently being modeled by the state of Virginia, may be an optimal way to get high-quality health care services to some of those in need for the least amount of money. Should more states adopt this approach, free clinics would be able to expand their ability to provide medical care to the uninsured and underinsured.

DEMOGRAPHIC CHANGES IN THE UNITED STATES

Among the key demographic changes that are likely to occur in the United States in the coming years, two are likely to have the greatest impact on free clinics: the increasing number of people age sixty and over and the increasing number of immigrants and political refugees.

The Aging of the Population

The graying of the American population will have a profound impact on the health care system, on Medicare, and on the need for free clinics. While life span (the maximum number of years of life) has increased only marginally in recent decades, life expectancy (the average number of years of life) has continued to increase. More people than ever are living past sixty-five, and the fastest-growing age group in the country is comprised of those age eighty-five and older. This means that more people—and an increasingly large percentage of the population—are living during the part of life when health problems mount, when the use of medical services is greatest, and when the demand for pharmaceuticals is highest. As baby boomers reach these older years, more of them will expect to draw upon Medicare, yet there will be a proportionately smaller percentage of the population working and paying in to the Medicare program. This is a problem for which Congress has failed to develop a long-term solution.

The obvious consequences of this demographic change are that the age for receiving Medicare benefits may increase, the percentage of one's medical care paid for by Medicare may decrease, or both. In addition, as reimbursement levels to health care providers fail to keep up with cost-of-living increases (or fall further behind), an increasing number of providers may refuse to see Medicare patients or will only see them if the patients pay something in addition to that covered by Medicare. If the age for Medicare eligibility increases and workers continue to retire in their early sixties, the number of years before they qualify for benefits will expand. As fewer employers provide health benefits for their retired workers, the medical needs of this post-sixty, pre-Medicare group of retirees could expand significantly.

Thus far, the most serious problem with Medicare is that it has not included a prescription drug benefit. This is the reason that Medicare enrollees have typically been able to see a provider and have this service partly or completely covered by Medicare but not receive any assistance in paying for medications. As the price of medications has continued to escalate rapidly, fewer and fewer enrollees have been able to pay for them. This is the reason that free clinic after free clinic reports that Medicare patients often forgo needed medication or that senior couples covered by Medicare often rotate taking a medication because they cannot afford to purchase it for both. While some seniors have purchased their own prescription drug policy, about one in four seniors has absolutely no coverage, and as many as 30 percent more have inadequate coverage.

In 2004, Congress passed a limited Medicare drug benefit. This drug benefit may be viewed from different perspectives. On the one hand, it breaks new territory by acknowledging the necessity of the federal government, through the Medicare program, assisting seniors in the purchase of medications—that is, there is symbolic importance. The dollars made available for seniors to make medication purchases will be helpful and, in some cases, may make the difference in being able or not being able to purchase the drug. But, on the other hand, the number of dollars made available fall far short of covering the need. The legislation includes no cap on drug price increases, so as the price of pharmaceuticals continues to jump, the actual out-of-pocket dollars needed by seniors to purchase drugs may change very little. Many analysts believe that the Medicare drug benefit will fall far short of meeting the need in the short term and fall even further short with each passing year. It is likely that the aggregate medical care needs of seniors will increase rapidly in the coming years, and that will require free clinics to make a determination of the extent to which they can offer continued or expanded service to this group.

Most free clinics do not now see patients if they have any form of health insurance, including Medicare. However, some provide free medications to Medicare patients. Because drugs represent the major expense at many free clinics, decisions about eligibility for medication assistance will continue to be very difficult. A comprehensive Medicare prescription drug benefit would have resolved this problem for seniors, but the bill passed ensures that it will continue to be an issue and possibly even grow in importance.

The Increase in the Immigrant and Refugee Populations

Never has it been so clear that the United States cannot isolate itself from the rest of the world. Most of the immigrants and political refugees (most legally documented but some not) entering the United States each year are very poor upon their arrival, enter living situations that are not healthy, experience serious acute and chronic illnesses, and do not have any form of health insurance. Many depend on free health clinics for their health care services. Many, many free clinics in the country—in the Northeast, Midwest, Southeast, heartland, Southwest, and Far West and in large, medium-sized, and small cities and towns have experienced a significant increase in recent years in their number of Hispanic patients. In most large cities, free clinics have Spanish-speaking staff members to assist in translation. In smaller cities and towns, where it is less likely to have a staff member who is fluent in Spanish, free clinics sometimes use community volunteers—often area college students majoring in Spanish—to assist with translation.

Recently arrived immigrants and refugees—especially those who do not speak English—often have a very difficult time applying for and obtaining community services for which they are eligible. This is one reason that most free clinics go beyond the provision of medical care and attempt to serve as a liaison with other services in the community. Free clinic staff and volunteers work closely with these patients to help them negotiate the system and to try to ensure that they have adequate shelter, food, and clothing. For undocumented immigrants, who typically are not eligible for the same array of services and who often are very fearful of making any contact with agencies or organizations, the task for the free clinic is greater and more complex. But the free clinic may be all that stands between these individuals—adults and children—and suffering from health problems that can be cured.

Dick Surrusco, MD, one of the founders of the Bradley Free Clinic and an emergency room physician, sees a very important role for free clinics in refugee resettlement.

> Free clinics are going to have to be identified as safety nets whose role is going to have to expand not only to access to medical and dental care but also access to psychiatric care and to play a critical role in the resettlement of immigrants. I think as we have more and more refugee resettlement evolving that free clinics are going to have to step up to the plate and become an integral part of that resettlement. I can tell you, as an emergency room physician, that the most nightmarish cases that I have had in the last five years have been with refugees who have arrived without English language skills, without resources, and with unbelievable health problems. The medical community is trying its best to accommodate these individuals, but we need an interface there—some way for these folks to be prepared to enter into the private sector. Our physicians will accept them into their practices—they do and they will—but in order to facilitate and coordinate the care that they receive, the free clinic needs to be involved in the transition.

Most analysts anticipate that the number of immigrants and refugees allowed to enter the United States each year will increase in the coming years as conditions in many countries deteriorate. If numbers stay where they are or increase, free clinics will be called upon to be an increasing factor in helping take care of their health care needs.

CORPORATE, FOUNDATION, AND PUBLIC SUPPORT

The sources from which free clinics draw funding raise difficult questions. One side of the issue, a strength of free clinics historically has been the fact that they have received most of their funds from within their own community. This has contributed to the special pride that many communities have in the free clinic and to the sense of identification the clinic has with the community. It has distinguished free clinics from public health departments, which typically receive much of their funding from the state, and from community action agencies, which receive funding from the federal government. Relying on community funding has, perhaps, contributed to the image or nature of the clinic in a way that has encouraged some individuals to come forward as volunteers. Many free clinics believe that their community base has facilitated in-kind contributions such as the willingness of hospitals to provide testing and other services for free clinic patients at no charge.

On the other hand, as much as free clinics contribute in their communities, there is widespread recognition that they are filling the health care needs for only part of the uninsured and the working poor and, in some cases, for other groups with glaring medical needs. The record of community fund-raising of free clinics has been rather astounding, yet with all of that, free clinics have been able to take care of only part of the need. With health care being so expensive, and health care costs continuing to rise so dramatically, it is uncertain that existing free clinics can expand significantly or that communities with one clinic will be able to add more. Several free clinic directors identify the biggest frustration in their job as being the inability to offer services to all of those truly in need.

> The number of people needing our services keeps getting greater. As long as we can keep this volunteer model going, we'll be just fine, but what if doctors say that they are doing all that they can do? We are totally dependent on the good will of the volunteers providing service and the institutions supporting us. If a crunch comes, and those institutions say that they can't help anymore, that it is too costly, then you are back to not having any way to get care to people. I've heard some legislators address the problem by saying that they are sure that free clinics are taking care of the problem. But we are taking care of not even the tip of the iceberg. Every time that sixty people walk in our door, sixty more could walk in behind them, and sixty more behind them, and we still wouldn't be helping everybody. So this is not the right way to serve all of those with needs even though we serve very well some of the people with needs. (Jean Lee, Executive Director, Free Medical Clinic of Northern Shenandoah Valley, Winchester, Virginia)

> Some days, our door is open for four or five minutes, and our clinic is full to capacity. (Leigh Ann Surgent, RN, St. Anthony Free Medical Clinic, San Francisco, California)

> Are we meeting all of the needs of those who are falling between the cracks of the health care system? No, but we are doing a good job of meeting the needs of those whom we are serving. (Jane Zwiers, Executive Director, Kalamazoo Free Clinic, Kalamazoo, Michigan)

> The biggest frustration is the realization that the need outweighs the resources, and that is hard. It is hard for me to tell people that we are so sorry, but we can't see them today—that we are already seeing as many patients as we possibly can. My husband jokingly tells me that I have a "fix-it" personality. If someone has a problem, get out of my way, and let me fix it. It has been hard to realize that I can't fix it for everybody. I have to focus and say that I haven't fixed it for everybody, but I have helped some. We try to do whatever we can whenever we can, but we have had to limit the number of times that patients can come to the clinic, so that we can get more people in to be seen. (Sandy Motley, Executive Director, Davidson Medical Ministries Clinic, Inc., Lexington, North Carolina)

I think free clinics are a partial solution to the problem and are designed, frankly, as a temporary solution. I am still in awe that in the richest nation in the world, we have so many people without access to health care. It is ludicrous when you look at the amount of dollars spent on other things. I think the free clinics can do better, however, if they are willing to reinvent themselves, and I'll give you an example. The mission statement of most free clinics is to provide care for the working poor. However, there are many people on Medicare whose needs are not being met who do not qualify as the working poor. I think we have a false sense of what public assistance means in terms of dollars. I think we have a false sense of what a disability check means in terms of dollars. I think we have a false sense of what entitlement programs are really delivering. So free clinic services are often refused to Medicare and Medicaid patients. I understand the economics that expanding the borders of who can be seen could reduce the services available to our primary population, the working poor. However, I think if clinics will be open enough to reinvent themselves in terms of funding and to look at funding sources that they have been reluctant to consider because of control issues, then I think we will be able to get a more global safety net. And, if not eliminating the holes in the safety net, then reducing it to a fine mesh. (Richard Surrusco, MD, an emergency room physician and one of the founders of the Bradley Free Clinic, Roanoke, Virginia)

The three most logical sources for additional funding are corporations, foundations, and government support including entitlement programs. There are many examples already in which free clinics have sought financial support from the corporate and private foundation sectors. For example, free clinics in Virginia are quick to acknowledge the importance of financial support from the Anthem Corporation (formerly Trigon, formerly Blue Cross Blue Shield of Virginia). Its grants to assist communities in starting a free clinic and its grants in supporting existing clinics are very important reasons for the large number of clinics in Virginia and for their financial stability. Grants from the Kate B. Reynolds Charitable Trust and the Duke Endowment and now the Blue Cross and Blue Shield of North Carolina Foundation have been extremely helpful to free clinics in North Carolina and have made it another state with widespread free clinic services. Many free clinics and free clinic state associations owe their start to the Robert Wood Johnson Foundation–sponsored Volunteers in Health Care. Funding from these and other corporate and private foundation sources clearly has enabled free clinics to serve more of their target population. The question is to what extent can foundation support be further tapped. Are there corporations or foundations in other states that will adopt free clinics as a special project? As the number of free clinics expands in states that already have support, will funders add to their contributions or simply divide them into more and smaller pieces?

A small but increasing number of free clinics now also receive public funding reimbursements. In some cases, these are direct allocations from the local government to assist free clinics in helping to meet the health care needs of people in the community. In some cases, state governments now allocate funds directly to free clinics or channel funds to individual clinics through the state association (as is done in Virginia) or through a state department (as is done in West Virginia). Some free clinics now apply for federal grant money and have established sizable programs, usually with a specific focus such as HIV prevention and care. Some clinics have asked whether refusing to be reimbursed by programs such as Medicare and Medicaid ultimately is in the clinic's best interest. But would receiving such funds dramatically change the essence of free clinics? Would the community base of support erode if federal funds became significant in a clinic's overall budget? What would be the difference between a free clinic and a community health clinic?

The Los Angeles Free Clinic is an example of a free clinic that has widely expanded its funding sources to include government contracts. The rationale has been that the needs are so great that the clinic must avail itself of all possible funding sources. There is recognition that the bureaucracy necessary to carry out these funded activities could alter the nature of the clinic, and there has been determination not to let this happen. But it is an important change.

As the need increases and the requirements increase to provide services through regulatory agencies, through contractors, through foundations, the needs have changed. We are in a position now that you can no longer just rely on fund-raising—you have to rely on contracts with the county, contracts with the state, contracts with the federal government, and it has dramatically changed the grassroots type of financial support that we used to rely on. It is changing the financial structure without hopefully changing the core mission. (Joseph Dunn, Ph.D., Executive Director, The Los Angeles Free Clinic, Los Angeles, California)

From my perspective, providing the care to our patients is the easy part. Seeing patients, talking to them about health issues, dispensing medications, providing as much access as you can, getting people in the door, that's not as hard as the paperwork and compliance with all of the regulations. A part of me longs for the days when I could recruit some doctors to come over, see patients in a broom closet, and just feel good about what we are doing. I miss that. It is not like it was in the sixties through the eighties. . . . When you start taking government dollars and government contracts, it has to change the nature of your organization. But I still think that a percentage of what we are doing is trying innovative ways of providing health care to the medically indigent. I think that is what distinguishes us—that we do have some unrestricted dollars that we can use to try new things—like a petri dish for exploring and overcoming the challenge of getting care to the poor. As an example, we recently were able to start an integrative medicine program that includes voluntary acupuncture, chiropractic, and other alternatives for our patients. (Susan Mandel, MD, Medical Director, Los Angeles Free Clinic, Los Angeles, California)

Thus, an important decision for free clinics individually and collectively will be how to raise sufficient money to add to the number of free clinics, how to maintain and increase the level of services offered in already existing clinics, and how to do this while maintaining the spirit of free clinics and not succumbing to bureaucratic overload. Clinics could stay at their current level and be contributing an enormous amount to millions of the working poor and other vulnerable groups. But with the needs being great already and likely increasing, there will be constant desire to find ways to do more.

DEVELOPMENT OF FREE CLINIC ASSOCIATIONS AND SUPPORTING ORGANIZATIONS

A fourth major factor that will impact the future course of free health clinics is the development and success of programs and collective organizations focused on the medically indigent. Four of the most important of these programs are: (1) state and regional free clinic associations; (2) the National Free Clinic Association; (3) long-standing groups that directly support free clinics such as Volunteers in Health Care, Volunteers in Medicine, and the National Free Clinic Foundation; and (4) alternative volunteer-based organizational formats for serving the medically indigent.

State and Regional Free Clinic Associations

In a relatively short amount of time, state and regional free clinic associations have established a very strong presence and are almost universally praised for the benefits that they have brought to clinics. Clinics that are members of state or regional associations provide glowing reports of the increased opportunities for networking, the value of shared resources, the inspirational lift of interacting with others in a shared cause, fund-raising benefits, and programmatic benefits. These associations are largely organization-based, that is, their primary focus is on assisting each of the individual free clinics to become stronger. Some of the associations also foresee opportunities for lobbying for the free clinic cause and making an impact on legislation. There have been some early successes, and some see these initiatives as a logical outgrowth of concern for the medically indigent. But policy-related initiatives also have the potential to be more controversial given the fact that not all of the people devoted to free clinics share views about specific health-related policies. Nevertheless, the state and regional associations have gained strong support. As the number of free clinics increases nationally and the free clinic movement takes hold in states that previously had little free clinic presence, it is likely that additional state and regional associations will emerge. In turn, that will help to create stronger individual clinics.

The National Association of Free Clinics

It is still very early in the life history of the National Association of Free Clinics. Based on the demise of the National Free Clinic Council in the early 1970s and the reluctance thereafter of many clinic people to think in terms of a national association, the complexities of developing a successful national association are clear. At this point, the NAFC has incorporated, created an organizational infrastructure, met its interim membership goals, developed a Web site, and enlarged networking, education, and information sharing on a national level. Work continues in gaining the support of additional individual clinics and free clinic advocates. Making the association a strong voice for free clinics and for the patients served by free clinics is an ambitious goal. If that can be accomplished, the role of free clinics in the overall health care system will be strengthened, and the medically indigent will have a new, powerful voice to speak on their behalf.

Long-Standing Groups Supporting Free Clinics

It is common for social movements and need-targeted, volunteer-based services to develop like limbs on a tree—that is, many types and many configurations of organizations develop. While they are united by a common cause, organizations develop differently, have different foci, and have different identities. Such is the case with free health clinics. The Volunteers in Health Care program continues to provide data and services to free clinics and to assist in the development of free clinics, Volunteers in Medicine continues to assist in clinic start-up, and the Free Clinic Foundation assists in the provision of data and with assistance to communities starting a new free clinic. The California clinics, including those in Haight-Ashbury, Los Angeles, Venice, and (though it is a very different model) Berkeley, continue to be a clinic focal point as are the rapidly increasing number of state and regional associations. The National Association of Free Clinics is gaining a stronger foothold. The establishment of new free clinics has never occurred at so rapid a pace.

While it is likely that all of these activity centers will continue to be visible forces in the free clinic movement, it will also be interesting to monitor the extent to which free clinics will be able to speak with a united voice. As free clinics increase in number and visibility, it will be natural for those outside the free clinic community to ask who is in the best position to represent the needs and interests of free clinics and the patients they serve. The organizational map of free clinics and their chief spokespersons will certainly influence the ultimate role that free clinics play within the health care system. The primary issue rests with what some consider to be the national association's strongest asset and others consider to be the main concern: the extent to which it will be a strong political lobbying force.

Alternative Volunteer-Based Organizational Formats
for Serving the Medically Indigent

Since 1995, a new organizational format—Project Access (PA)—has come into being with the aim of expanding the nation's safety net for the uninsured. In the fall of 1994, the Buncombe County (Asheville, North Carolina) Medical Society received a one-year community health planning grant from the Robert Wood Johnson Foundation and subsequent grants from the Janirve Foundation, the Community Foundation of Western North Carolina, and the Kate B. Reynolds Charitable Trust to initiate and develop the BCMS Project Access. The ambitious goal of Project Access was to provide access to health care for every low-income, uninsured person within the county (about 15,000 of the county's 190,000 residents).

As designed, Project Access enables uninsured people who meet a specified level of eligibility guidelines to receive both a Project Access identification card (that entitles them to free or reduced-cost care from physicians and hospitals who agree to volunteer with the program) and a prescription card (that entitles them to free or reduced-cost medications). Typically, family or individual income must be below 200 percent of the federally established poverty level. In 2004, this was $17,960 for an individual, $24,240 for a couple or single parent and child, and $30,520 for a three-person household. Primary care physicians and specialists agree to see up to a specified number of PA patients per year (in Buncombe County, primary care physicians see up to ten patients each per year, and specialists up to twenty). The foundation of the program is a large pool of physicians and hospitals that agree to donate services. In Buncombe County almost 500 physicians (85 percent of local physicians), all of the area hospitals, area pharmacies (which provide medications at reduced—sometimes less than wholesale—prices), and a health insurer (providing free claims tracking services) have joined the program, and they provide more than $4 million in medical services free each year. The cost for medications (in Buncombe County, about $300,000 per year) is provided by the local government.

The Project Access program is designed so that it can work on a cooperative basis with and utilize free clinics and other providers of services for low-income persons. In most communities, the program has recognized that certain features of free clinics—such as on-site comprehensive services, being a liaison with other community services, assistance with pharmaceutical companies' indigent assistance programs, integrated health education programs, evening hours, and the special ambience of volunteer-driven services—are not easily duplicated in most private physicians' offices. Therefore, PA patients may choose to be seen—and many do—at the free clinic instead of a physician's office. The Asheville-Buncombe Community Christian Ministries Free Clinic works with Project Access and sees many PA patients.

Community health leaders in Buncombe County believe that they have created a successful safety net for the uninsured. "We believe that everybody has a right to health care, and we have set up a system in our community that allows that to happen," says Suzanne Landis, MD and M.P.H., a family practice physician in Asheville who helped to start the Buncombe County PA program (Adams 2002).

In 1999, the Buncombe County Medical Society established a cooperative relationship with the U.S. Bureau of Primary Care to assist other communities throughout the country in creating a Project Access program. By early 2004, PA programs had been initiated in Dallas County (Dallas, Texas), Emanuel County (Swainsboro, Georgia), Greenville County (Greenville, South Carolina), Guilford County (Guilford, North Carolina), Marquette County (Marquette, Michigan), Pitt County (Greenville, North Carolina), Pittsylvania County (Danville, Virginia), Sedgwick County (Wichita, Kansas), Shawnee County (Topeka, Kansas), Travis County (Austin, Texas), Wake County (Raleigh, North Carolina), and Wautaga County (Boone, North Carolina). In addition, more than fifty other communities around the country are currently in the process of starting a PA program. Not every program is structured in exactly the same way. For example, in some communities diagnostic services may be covered but not hospital services.

Assessment studies have documented program benefits. There is emphasis on preventive care, so that the uninsured do not have to wait for medical crises to get care. Use of the hospital emergency room for nonemergent care has decreased noticeably. Physicians are able to volunteer within the scope of their practice and to treat PA patients without having to follow the dictates of managed care. Most importantly, more than 80 percent of residents who have used the system report that their health is either better or much better than when they first enrolled in the program (West 1999).

When Project Access enters a community with an existing free clinic, development of a cooperative relationship is extremely important. Both programs seek volunteers from the provider community, and both rely on donated services from hospitals and other medical organizations. The chance for misunderstandings, divided community loyalties, and even competition exists—none of which would be to the best interest of patients. Perhaps an ideal model is that established in Roanoke, Virginia, in which the long-established Bradley Free Clinic oversees the PA program. That enables complete coordination of the two programs and enables them to speak with a united voice in community presentations and in interaction with medical providers.

CONCLUSION

The need for available medical care services for the uninsured and underinsured is already great and will likely increase substantially both in the short term and in the long term. Will free clinics be able to sustain and increase the current level of services? Will the number of free clinics continue to increase? Will existing free clinics be able to expand their services? Will more and more volunteers come forward? Will additional communities take the initiative in investigating the possibility of creating a free clinic? Will additional corporations and foundations make a major commitment to free clinics? Will free clinics become a stronger voice advocating for people who now go without needed medical services?

Even now, it is safe to say that rarely have so many done so much good for so many people with so little fanfare. Free health clinic staff and volunteers understand that they now provide access to medical care for only a relatively small portion of the nation's medically unserved, but that small portion equates to millions of people each year who receive high-quality care that is delivered with respect and compassion from incredibly dedicated staff members and volunteers. Free clinics exemplify grassroots efforts of communities to address the unmet medical needs of those in their population who do not have access to the private care system. The clinics may not yet have transformed the nation's overall medical care system, but they have genuinely had a transforming effect on those who deliver care there, on the communities in which they are located, and, most importantly, on the individuals and families who receive needed medical care.

> The free clinic is more than a place to receive health care. It benefits not only those who come there for care but also those who deliver the care. In a broader frame of reference, it helps to transform the entire town into a community. Think about this in 1,000 communities, or better yet, in 10,000. We could transform communities across the country. We could change the way that medicine is practiced in the United States. (Jack McConnell, MD, founder, Volunteers in Medicine Clinic, Hilton Head, South Carolina)

Bibliography

Abramson, Randi, MD, Bread for the City/Zacchaeus Free Clinic, Washington, DC, personal interview with the author, April 5, 2002.

Adams, Damon. "Project Access: Opening the Door to Health Care." *Amednews.com,* January 21, 2002. www.ama-assn.org/amednews/2002/01/21/prsa0121.htm.

Alford, Robert. *Bureaucracy and Participation: Political Culture in Four Wisconsin Cities.* Chicago: Rand McNally, 1969.

Alliance for Health Reform. "Health Care Coverage in America: Understanding the Issues and Proposed Solutions." www.CovertheUninsured.org.

Amodia, Diana, MD, Haight-Ashbury Free Clinics, Inc., San Francisco, California, personal interview with the author, August 15, 2001.

Anderson, Gerard, and Peter S. Hussey. "Comparing Health Care System Performance in OECD Countries." *Health Affairs* 20 (2001): 219–32.

Arenas, Janet, CommunityHealth, Chicago, Illinois, personal interview with the author, August 15, 2002.

Avner, Estelle Nichols, Bradley Free Clinic, Inc., Roanoke, Virginia, personal interview with the author, 2002.

Aycoth, Shirley, RN, Mercer Healthright, Inc., Bluefield, West Virginia, personal interview with the author, May 6, 2002.

Bacon, Franklin, Charlottesville Free Clinic, Charlottesville, Virginia, personal interview with the author, November 13, 2001.

Baird, Macon, Open Door Clinic of Alamance County, Burlington, North Carolina, personal interview with the author, November 7, 2001.

Barker, Anne, RN, Health Alliance for Patients in Need, Columbia, Maryland, personal interview with the author, April 4, 2002.

Barry, Patricia. "Chasing Drugs: Millions Cut Corners." *AARP Bulletin* 44 (2003): 3–6.

Bartolome, John, St. Anthony Free Medical Clinic, San Francisco, California, personal interview with the author, August 14, 2001.

Basart, Ann, Information and Referral Collective, Berkeley Free Clinic, Berkeley, California, personal interview with the author, August 16, 2001.

Baugh, David K., Penelope L. Pine, Steve Blackwell, and Gary Ciborowski. "Medicaid Prescription Drug Spending in the 1990s: A Decade of Change." *Health Care Financing Review* 25 (2004): 5–23.

Becker, Penny E., and Pawan H. Dhingra. "Religious Involvement and Volunteering: Implications for Civil Society." *Sociology of Religion* 62 (2001): 315–35.

Beckner, James, Fan Free Clinic, Inc., Richmond, Virginia, personal interview with the author, November 12, 2001.

Bibeau, Daniel L., Martha L. Taylor, John C. Rife, and Keith A. Howell. "Reaching the Poor with Health Promotion Through Community Free Clinics." *American Journal of Health Promotion* 12 (1997): 87–89.

Bice, Carla, RN, MPA, St. Joseph Health Center, South Bend, Indiana, personal interview with the author, August 12, 2002.

Bliziotes, Terri, RN, West Virginia Health Right, Inc., Charleston, West Virginia, personal interview with the author, May 6, 2002.

Bridges, Marilynn, Free Clinic of Franklin County, Inc., Rocky Mount, Virginia, personal interview with the author, June 26, 2002.

Bureau of Labor Statistics. "Volunteering in the United States, 2003." www.bls.gov/cps.

Buenzli, Cam, RN, Healthnet of Janesville, Inc., Janesville, Wisconsin, personal interview with the author, August 14, 2002.

Caldarella, Maggie, RN, Bradley Free Clinic, Inc., Roanoke, Virginia, personal interview with the author, 2002.

Carnevale, Anthony P., and Stephen J. Rose. "Low Earners: Who Are They? Do They Have a Way Out?" In *Low Wage Workers in the New Economy*, edited by Richard Kazis and Marc S. Miller, 45–65. Washington, DC: Urban Institute Press, 2001.

Canton Community Clinic. *Canton Community Clinic—A Community-Based Solution to the Former Problem of Nearly Non-Existent Primary Health Care for the Poor in Stark County*. Canton, OH: Canton Community Clinic, 2001.

Clark, Harry W. "How Relevant is the Free Clinic Movement to Black People." *Journal of Social Issues* 30 (1974): 67–72.

Clark, Sandra, MD, Robert Nixon Medical Clinic, Chapel Hill, North Carolina, personal interview with the author, November 5, 2001.

Consumer Reports. "The Unraveling of Health Insurance." July 2002, 48–53.

Cornelius, Linda, Augusta Regional Free Clinic, Fishersville, Virginia, personal interview with the author, October 4, 2001.

Cowgill, Sandy, Will-Grundy Medical Clinic, Joliet, Illinois, personal interview with the author, August 13, 2002.

Cruise, Mark, Virginia Association of Free Clinics and National Association of Free Clinics, Richmond, Virginia, personal interviews with the author, November 12, 2001.

Cutler, David M. *Your Money or Your Life: Strong Medicine for America's Health Care System*. New York: Oxford University Press, 2004.

Cutler, Rebecca. "Chicagoans of the Year—Our Heroes: Dr. Serafina Garella." *Chicago*, January 2001, 69.

Dedrick, Patricia. "Survey Examines Medically Uninsured." *Birmingham Post Herald*, March 8, 2003.

Dillow, Judy, First Baptist Church of North Charleston Medical Clinic, North Charleston, South Carolina, personal interview with the author, September 13, 2001.

Doll, William. "Whatever Happened to the 60s Free Clinics?" *New Physician*, April 1985, 8–11.

Donelan, Karen, Robert J. Blendon, Cathy Schoen, Karen Davis, and Katherine Binns. "The Cost of Health System Change: Public Discontent in Five Nations." *Health Affairs* 18 (1999): 206–16.

Downin, Jeffrey, Community Free Clinic, Hagerstown, Maryland, personal interview with the author, October 5, 2001.

Drury, Sandra, Free Clinic of Reidsville and Vicinity, Inc., Reidsville, North Carolina, personal interview with the author, November 5, 2001.

Dunn, Joseph, PhD, The Los Angeles Free Clinic, Los Angeles, California, personal interview with the author, August 22, 2001.

Elena. "History and Politics of the Berkeley Free Clinic." Unpublished paper. 1998.

Elliott, Margaret, Crisis Control Ministry, Winston-Salem, North Carolina, personal interview with the author, November 6, 2001.

Elmore, Lee, RN, North Coast Health Ministry, Lakewood, Ohio, personal interview with the author, May 2, 2002.

Enigk, Debra, Mercer Healthright, Inc., Bluefield, West Virginia, personal interview with the author, May 6, 2002.

Flowers, Casey, RN, Free Clinic of Reidsville and Vicinity, Inc., Reidsville, North Carolina, personal interview with the author, November 5, 2001.

Forer, Liz, Venice Family Clinic, Venice, California, telephone interview with the author, October 11, 2002.

Free Clinic Foundation of America. *National Free Clinic Directory*. 4th ed. Roanoke, VA: The Bradley Free Clinic, 2000.

Free Clinics of the Great Lakes Region. www.fcglr.net.

Freeman, Jo. *Waves of Protest: Social Movements of the Sixties and Seventies*. Essex: Longman Group, 1983.

Friedman, Carol, Farque Ahmed, Adele Franks, Tom Weatherup, Marsha Manning, April Vance, and Betsy Thompson. "Association Between Health Insurance Coverage of Office Visit and Cancer Screening Among Women." *Medical Care* 40 (2002): 1060–67.

Frumkin, Peter. *On Being Nonprofit: A Conceptual and Policy Primer*. Cambridge, MA: Harvard University Press, 2002.

Fuller, Diane, RN, North Coast Health Ministry, Lakewood, Ohio, personal interview with the author, May 2, 2002.

Galbis, Ricardo. "The Free Clinics: Approach to Alienated Youth." In *The Free Clinic: A Community Approach to Health Care and Drug Abuse,* edited by David E. Smith, David J. Bentel, and Jerome L. Schwartz, 120–26. Beloit, WI: Stash Press, 1971.

Garvin, John, MD, Bradley Free Clinic, Inc., Roanoke, Virginia, personal interview with the author, 2002.

Giled, Sherry, and Sarah E. Little. "The Uninsured and the Benefits of Medical Practice." *Health Affairs* 22 (2003): 210–19.

Gleason, Thomas, St. Anthony Foundation, San Francisco, California, personal interview with the author, August 14, 2001.

Goretzka, Pastor Keith, First Baptist Church of North Charleston Medical Clinic, North Charleston, South Carolina, personal interview with the author, September 13, 2001.

Gottlieb, Karen, Americares Free Clinics, New Canaan, Connecticut, telephone interview with the author, September 17, 2002.

Halstead, Virginia Garza, Hollywood Sunset Free Clinic, Los Angeles, California, personal interview with the author, August 21, 2001.

Harrelson, Verle, The Free Medical Clinic, Columbia, South Carolina, personal interview with the author, September 11, 2001.

Harvey, William M. "Special Problems of Free Clinics Serving Minority Communities." *Journal of Social Issues* 30 (1974): 61–66.

Hayner, Greg, DPharm., Haight-Ashbury Free Clinics, Inc., San Francisco, California, personal interview with the author, August 15, 2001.

Helfman, Frances, Los Angeles Free Clinic, Los Angeles, California, personal interview with the author, August 21, 2001.

Hiller, Marty, Free Clinic of Greater Cleveland, Cleveland, Ohio, personal interview with the author, May 2, 2002.

Hunt, Ann Marie, RN, Canton Community Clinic, Canton, Ohio, personal interview with the author, May 3, 2002.

Husain, Sairah, Berkeley Free Clinic, Berkeley, California, personal interview with the author, August 16, 2001.

Hutchinson, Regina, Mercy Medicine Clinic, Florence, South Carolina, personal interview with the author, September 12, 2001.

Idol, Pamela, RN, Davidson Medical Ministries Clinic, Inc., Lexington, North Carolina, personal interview with the author, November 6, 2001.

Institute of Medicine. "Care Without Coverage: Too Little, Too Late." www.books.nap.edu/ html/care_without/reportbrief.pdf.

Jones, Karon, RN, Free Clinic of Franklin County, Inc., Rocky Mount, Virginia, personal interview with the author, June 26, 2002.

Judis, John. "The Spirit of '68: What Really Caused the Sixties." *New Republic* 219 (1998): 20–26.

Kaiser Commission on Medicaid and the Uninsured. "The Uninsured: A Primer—Key Facts About Americans Without Health Insurance." www.kff.org/uninsured/loader.cfm?url= commonspot/security/getfile.cfm@PageID=29345.

Kelleher, Kevin, MD, Bradley Free Clinic, Inc., Roanoke, Virginia, personal interview with the author, 2002.

Klandermans, Bert, and Dirk Oegema. "Potentials, Networks, Motivations, and Barriers: Steps Towards Participation in Social Movements." *American Sociological Review* 52 (1987): 519–31.

Kroman, David, Berkeley Free Clinic, Berkeley, California, personal interview with the author, 2001.

Kucinic, Carolyn, Will-Grundy Medical Clinic, Joliet, Illinois, personal interview with the author, August 13, 2002.

Lam, Pui-Yan. "As the Flocks Gather: How Religion Affects Voluntary Association Participation." *Journal for the Scientific Study of Religion* 41 (2002): 405–22.

Landes, Juanita, Augusta Regional Free Clinic, Fishersville, Virginia, personal interview with the author, October 4, 2001.

Lassey, Marie L., William R. Lassey, and Martin J. Jinks. *Health Care Systems Around the World.* Upper Saddle River, NJ: Prentice Hall, 1997.

Lee, Jean, Free Medical Clinic of Northern Shenandoah Valley, Winchester, Virginia, personal interview with the author, October 4, 2001.

Lee, Stephen, MD, Los Angeles, California, personal interview with the author, August 21, 2001.

Leichter, Howard M. *A Comparative Approach to Policy Analysis: Health Care Policy in Four Nations.* Cambridge: Cambridge University Press, 1979.

Los Angeles Times. "Free For All," Sunday Profile, July 13, 1997. Reprinted at www.lafreeclinic.org/who_we_are/los_angeles_times.htm.

Mack, Pam, Health Alliance for Patients in Need, Columbia, Maryland, personal interview with the author, April 4, 2002.

Madaeu, Donna, Free Medical Clinic of Northern Shenandoah Valley, Winchester, Virginia, personal interview with the author, October 4, 2001.

Mandel, Susan A., MD, The Los Angeles Free Clinic, Los Angeles, California, personal interview with the author, August 21, 2001.

McConnell, Jack, MD, Volunteers in Medicine Clinic, Hilton Head Island, South Carolina, telephone interview with the author, October 4, 2002.

McConnell, Jack B., MD. *Circle of Caring: The Story of the Volunteers in Medicine Clinic.* Englewood, CO: The Estes Park Institute, 1998.

McCray, Fred, Augusta Regional Free Clinic, Fishersville, Virginia, personal interview with the author, October 4, 2001.

McCray, Shirley, Augusta Regional Free Clinic, Fishersville, Virginia, personal interview with the author, October 4, 2001.

McDavid, Kathleen, Thomas G. Tucker, Andrew Sloggett, and Michael P. Coleman. "Cancer Survival in Kentucky and Health Insurance Cover." *Archives of Internal Medicine* 163 (2003): 2135–44.

McHaley, Carol, DuPage Community Clinic, Wheaton, Illinois, personal interview with the author, August 13, 2002.

Michalski, Laura, CommunityHealth, Chicago, Illinois, personal interview with the author, August 15, 2002.

Mills, John, DPharm, North Carolina Association of Free Clinics, Winston-Salem, North Carolina, personal interview with the author, November 6, 2001.

Moore, Cynthia, FNP, Good Samaritan Clinic, Inc., Parkersburg, West Virginia, personal interview with the author, May 2, 2002.

Motley, Sandy, RN, Davidson Medical Ministries Clinic, Inc., Lexington, North Carolina, personal interview with the author, November 6, 2001.

Mullinax, Nadine, Community Free Clinic, Hagerstown, Maryland, personal interview with the author, October 5, 2001.

Nadkarni, Mohan N., and John T. Philbrick. "Free Clinics and the Uninsured: The Increasing Demands of Chronic Illness." *Journal of Health Care for the Poor and Underserved* 14 (2003): 165–74.

Nanus, Burt, and Stephen M. Dobbs. *Leaders Who Make a Difference: Essential Strategies for Meeting the Nonprofit Challenge.* San Francisco: Jossey-Bass Publishers, 1999.

Nathaniel, Alvita, NP, Mercer Healthright, Inc., Bluefield, West Virginia, personal interview with the author, May 6, 2002.

National Association of Free Clinics. www.nafclinics.org.

North Carolina Association of Free Clinics. www.ncfreeclinics.org.

———. "Blue Cross and Blue Shield of North Carolina Foundation Makes Historic Contribution to NC Free Clinics." *Free Clinic Happenings* 2 (2004): 1.

Padua, Tacy, Hollywood Sunset Free Clinic, Los Angeles, California, personal interview with the author, August 21, 2001.

Pierce, Glenn, ABCCM Medical Ministry, Asheville, North Carolina, personal interview with the author, June 25, 2002.

Powis, Neville. "The Human Be-In and the Hippy Revolution." www.rwninl/special/en/ html/031221be-in.html, 2003.

Price, Suzie, RN, Mercy Medicine Clinic, Florence, South Carolina, personal interview with the author, September 12, 2001.

Reiner-Good, Rachel, Hilltop Health Center, Valparaiso, Indiana, personal interview with the author, August 12, 2002.

Rhea, Randy, MD, Bradley Free Clinic, Inc., Roanoke, Virginia, personal interview with the author, 2002.

Riley, Eric, Canton Community Clinic, Canton, Ohio, personal interview with the author, May 3, 2002.

Riley, Trish, and Elizabeth Kilbreth. "Health Coverage in the States—Maine's Plan for Universal Access." *New England Journal of Medicine* 350 (2004): 330–32.

Rives, Tom, MD, Friendship House, Conway, South Carolina, personal interview with the author, September 13, 2001.

Roberson, Robin, Community Free Clinic, Hagerstown, Maryland, personal interview with the author, October 5, 2001.

Sadet, Andrea, Free Medical Clinic of Northern Shenandoah Valley, Winchester, Virginia, personal interview with the author, October 4, 2001.

Schiesl, Patricia, Health Care Network, Inc., Racine, Wisconsin, personal interview with the author, August 13, 2002.

Schriver, Melinda L. *No Health Insurance: It's Enough to Make You Sick.* Philadelphia, PA: American College of Physicians–American College of Internal Medicine, 1999.

Schwartz, Jerome L. 1971 "Preliminary Observations of Free Clinic." In *The Free Clinic: A Community Approach to Health Care and Drug Abuse,* edited by David E. Smith, David J. Bentel, and Jerome L. Schwartz, 144–206. Beloit, WI: Stash Press, 1971.

Sella, Becky, Friendship House, Conway, South Carolina, personal interview with the author, September 13, 2001.

Seymour, Richard B., MA, Haight-Ashbury Free Clinics, Inc., San Francisco, California, personal interview with the author, August 15, 2001.

Seymour, Richard B., and David E. Smith 1986. *The Haight Ashbury Free Medical Clinics: Still Free After All These Years.* San Francisco: Partisan Press.

Shapiro, Diana, Berkeley Free Clinic, Berkeley, California, personal interview with the author, August 16, 2001.

Sheridan, Suzanne, Rockbridge Area Free Clinic, Lexington, Virginia, personal interview with the author, November 13, 2001.

Shulman, Beth. *The Betrayal of Work: How Low-Wage Jobs Fail 30 Million Americans and Their Families.* New York: New Press, 2003.

Skaff, Vic, DDS, Bradley Free Clinic, Inc., Roanoke, Virginia, personal interview with the author, 2002.

Smith, David E., MD, Haight-Ashbury Free Clinics, Inc., San Francisco, California, personal interview with the author, August 15, 2001.

Smith, David E., David J. Bentel, and Jerome L. Schwartz. "Introduction." In *The Free Clinic: A Community Approach to Health Care and Drug Abuse,* edited by David E. Smith, David J. Bentel, and Jerome L. Schwartz, ix–xviii. Beloit, WI: Stash Press, 1971.

Snow, David A., Louis A. Zurcher, and Sheldon Ekland-Olson. "Social Networks and Social Movements: A Microstructural Approach to Differential Recruitment." *American Sociological Review* 45 (1980): 787–801.

Sparrow, Parker, RN, The Free Medical Clinic, Columbia, South Carolina, personal interview with the author, September 11, 2001.

State Health Access Data Assistance Center. www.shadac.umn.edu

Sturges, Clark S. *Doctor Dave.* Walnut Creek, CA: Devil Mountain Books, 1993.

Surgent, Leigh Ann, RN, St. Anthony Free Medical Clinic, San Francisco, California, personal interview with the author, August 14, 2001.

Surrusco, Richard, MD, Bradley Free Clinic, Inc., Roanoke, Virginia, personal interview with the author, 2002.

Tylenda, Barb, Health Care Network, Inc., Racine, Wisconsin, personal interview with the author, August 13, 2002.

Van Riper, Paige, The Los Angeles Free Clinic, Los Angeles, California, personal interview with the author, August 22, 2001.

Van Zoeren, Doug, MD, Washington Free Clinic, Washington, DC, personal interview with the author, August 4, 2002.

Vermont Coalition of Clinics for the Uninsured. www.vccu.net.

Virginia Association of Free Clinics. www.vafreeclinics.org.

Weiss, Gregory L. "Virginia's Free Medical Clinics: The Relationship Between Alternative Image and Community Support." *Virginia Social Science Journal* 14 (1980): 52–57.

———. "Adaptability and Change in Alternative Institutions: An Analysis of Free Health Clinics in the Southeastern United States." *Virginia Social Science Journal* 19 (1984): 22–28.

West, Kayla. "Buncombe County Medical Society Project Access." Buncombe Medical Society. www.projectaccessonline.org/health_outcome_study.html, 1999.

Weybright, Becky, Charlottesville Free Clinic, Charlottesville, Virginia, personal interview with the author, November 13, 2001.

White, Jeri, M.Ed., The Community Clinic of High Point, High Point, North Carolina, personal interview with the author, June 26, 2002.

White, Patricia Holmes, West Virginia Health Right, Inc., Charleston, West Virginia, personal interview with the author, May 6, 2002.

Wilcoxen, Carolyn, Good Samaritan Clinic, Inc., Parkersburg, West Virginia, personal interview with the author, May 2, 2002.

Wilson, John, and Thomas Janoski. "The Contribution of Religion to Volunteer Work." *Sociology of Religion* 56 (1995): 137–52.

Wood, Sheri, Kansas City Free Health Clinic, Kansas City, Missouri, telephone interview with the author, September 16, 2002.

Wrobel, Beth, Hilltop Health Center, Valparaiso, Indiana, personal interview with the author, August 12, 2002.

Wuthnow, Robert. "Mobilizing Civic Engagement: The Changing Impact of Religious Involvement." In *Civic Engagement in American Democracy,* edited by Theda Skocpol and Morris P. Fiorina, 331–63. Washington, DC: Brookings Institution Press, 1999.

Zwiers, Jane, RN, First Presbyterian Church Health Clinic, Kalamazoo, Michigan, telephone interview with the author, October 9, 2002.

Index

About the Author

Greg Weiss is professor of sociology at Roanoke College in Salem, Virginia. He has received several awards for teaching and scholarship, including a TIAA-CREF Outstanding Virginia Faculty Award in 2004 and the American Sociological Association Section on Teaching and Learning in Sociology Hans Mauksch Award for Distinguished Contributions to Teaching in 2005. He is coauthor with Lynne Lonnquist of *The Sociology of Health, Healing and Illness* (now in its fifth edition) and coauthor with Kerry Strand of *Experiencing Social Research*.